Ultrasmall lanthanide oxide nanoparticles for biomedical imaging and therapy

Related titles:

Implantable sensor systems for biomedical applications
(ISBN 978-1-84569-987-1)

Biosensors for medical applications
(ISBN 978-1-84569-935-2)

Biomaterials for cancer therapeutics
(ISBN 978-0-85709-664-7)

Woodhead Publishing Series in Biomaterial: Number 68

Ultrasmall lanthanide oxide nanoparticles for biomedical imaging and therapy

Gang Ho Lee, Yongmin Chang
and Tae-Jeong Kim

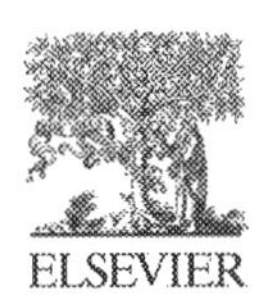

AMSTERDAM • BOSTON • CAMBRIDGE • HEIDELBERG • LONDON
NEW YORK • OXFORD • PARIS • SAN DIEGO
SAN FRANCISCO • SINGAPORE • SYDNEY • TOKYO
Woodhead Publishing is an imprint of Elsevier

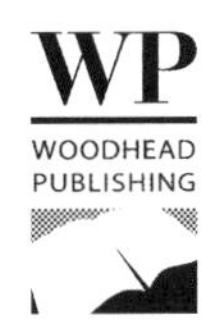

Woodhead Publishing is an imprint of Elsevier
80 High Street, Sawston, Cambridge, CB22 3HJ, UK
225 Wyman Street, Waltham, MA 02451, USA
Langford Lane, Kidlington, OX5 1GB, UK

British Library Cataloguing-in-Publication Data
A catalogue record for this book is available from the British Library

Library of Congress Control Number: 2014946710

ISBN 978-0-08100-066-3 (print)
ISBN 978-0-08100-069-4 (online)

For information on all Woodhead Publishing publications visit our website at http://store.elsevier.com/

Typeset by RefineCatch Limited, Bungay, Suffolk

Printed and bound in the United Kingdom

To my family:

Gang Ho Lee

Contents

List of figures and tables

Figures

Tables

List of abbrevations

ACK	Auger and Coster-Kronig
AOT	sodium bis(2-ethylhexyl) sulfosuccinate
ATP	adenosine-triphosphate
Au	gold
bcc	body-centered cubic
BNCT	boron neutron capture therapy
BPA	boronophenylalanine, $C_9H_{12}BNO_4$
BSA	bovine serum albumin
BSH	mercaptoundecahydro-dodecaborate-^{10}B or sodium borocaptate, $Na_2B_{12}H_{11}SH$
CT	computed tomography
2-D	two-dimensional
3-D	three-dimensional
DAPI	4′,6 diamidino-2-phenylindole
DEG	diethylene glycol
DLS	dynamic light scattering
Escherichia coli	*E. coli*
EDX	energy-dispersive X-ray spectrometer
EDS	energy-dispersive X-ray spectrometer
EELS	electron energy loss spectroscopy
EL4-Luc	lymphoma cells
FC	field-cooled

fcc	face-centered cubic
FDG	fluorodeoxyglucose
FI	fluorescent imaging
FT-IR	Fourier transform infrared
FWHM	full width at half maximum
^{157}Gd	Gadolimium-157
Gd_2O_3	gadolimium oxide
$Gd_2O(CO_3)_2.H_2O$	gadolinium carbonate hydrate
GdNCT	gadolimium neutron capture therapy
H_c	coercivity
ICPAES	inductively coupled plasma atomic emission spectrometer
KNU	Kyungpook National University
HAADF	high-angle annular dark-field imaging
hcp	hexagonal close packed
HRTEM	high resolution transmission electron microscope
HVEM	high voltage electron microscope
I	iodine
LDH	lactate dehydrogenase
Ln	lanthanide
Ln_2O_3	lanthanide oxide
$Ln(OH)_3$	lanthanide hydroxide
M-H	magnetization versus applied field
M-T	magnetization versus temperature
M_{NP}	net magnetic moment of a nanoparticle
MRI	magnetic resonance imaging
M_r	remanence
M_s	saturation magnetization
MTT	3-(4,5-dimethylthiazol-2-yl)-2,5-diphenyltetrazolium bromide

NAD^+	nicotinamide adenine dinucleotide
NADH	nicotinamide adenine dinucleotide hydrogen
NCT	neutron capture therapy
NGM	nematode growth medium
NIR	near infrared
NMOF	nanoscale metal organic framework
NSF	nephrogenic systemic fibrosis
Oe	oersted
PAA	poly acrylic acid
PBS	phosphate buffer saline
PEG	polyethylene glycol
PEI	polyethyleneimine
PET	positron emission tomography
PFA	paraformaldehyde
PL	photoluminescence
PVP	polyvinylpyrrolidone
PZT	piezoelectric transducer
r_1	longitudinal water proton relaxitivity
r_2	transverse water proton relaxitivity
QD	quantum dot
SPECT	single photon emission computed tomography
SPIO	superparamagnetic iron oxide
SQUID	superconducting quantum interference device
STA	Science and Technology Agency
STEM	scanning transmission electron microscope
SWNH	single-wall carbon nanohorn
SWNT	Signle-wall carbon nanotube
T_1	longitudinal water proton relaxation time

T_2	transverse water proton relaxation time
T_B	blocking temperature
T_C	Curie temperature
^{99m}Tc-HMPAO	hexamethylpropyleneamine oxime
^{99m}Tc-sestamibi	[methoxyisobutylisonitrile]$_6$
^{99m}Tc-tetrofosmin	[1,2-bis[di-(2-ethoxyethyl) phosphino]ethane]$_2$
T_N	Niel temperature
TEG	triethylene glycol
TEM	transmission electron microscope
TEOS	tetraethylorthosilicate
tetrazolium salt INT	2-(4-iodophenyl)-3-(4-nitrophenyl)-5-phenyl-2H-tetrazolium chloride
TGA	thermogravimetric analyzer
USI	ultrasound imaging
US-SWNT	ultra-short SWNT
UV	ultra-violet
W	tungsten
XRD	X-ray diffraction
ZFC	zero-field-cooled

Acknowledgments

There are many people whom I would like to thank. First of all, I would like to thank my family for their loving support. Without them, this book would never have been published. So it is to my family that this book is dedicated.

I would like to thank the talented students who have worked in my laboratory. This book is largely based on their hard work. I will remember them for their enthusiasm, persistence, and hard work.

I would like to thank the professors and scientists with whom I have worked so far in various projects in the fields of bioimaging, nanomedicine, and nanoscience.

Finally, I would like to thank Chandos Publishing and Woodhead Publishing for providing me with the opportunity to write this book.

Gang Ho Lee, PhD

Preface

Molecular imaging is a vital tool for diagnosis and treatment of disease. A variety of molecular imaging modalities have been developed so far. These include magnetic resonance imaging (MRI), X-ray computed tomography (CT), ultrasound imaging (USI), positron emission tomography (PET), single photon emission computed tomography (SPECT), and fluorescent imaging (FI).

Molecular imaging agents can be used to improve image quality. When applied to patients, molecular imaging agents should be, first of all, non-toxic. They should be completely excreted from the body through the renal system after imaging, unless they can be digested in the body through metabolic process. Until now, a variety of molecular imaging agents have been developed for clinical applications and are also under further development.

Although clinically applicable molecular imaging agents are mostly small molecules, enormous efforts have been paid to developing new imaging agents. There is no doubt that one of such candidates is a nanoparticle imaging agent as dealt with in this book. The primary reason for this would be the enhanced imaging properties of nanoparticles compared to molecular imaging agents.

This book focuses on ultrasmall lanthanide oxide nanoparticles, which have a variety of magnetic and optical properties. Therefore, they could be potential MRI contrast agents and FI agents. They also have high X-ray attenuation properties that could be used as CT contrast agents. Gadolinium (^{157}Gd) oxide nanoparticles also have a very large thermal neutron capture cross-section that could be used as a neutron capture therapy (NCT) agent against cancers. Due to these diverse properties, ultrasmall lanthanide oxide nanoparticles seem to be promising multifunctional materials for biomedical imaging and therapy. They are compact, robust, and stable because they are solid-state, which will be extremely useful for biomedical applications.

'Seeing is believing.' Seeing is the most reliable or least-doubt sense to convince us of the fact. Therefore, it may be true to say that medicine has developed with biomedical imaging.

I hope that this book will be useful for both students and scientists who are interested in molecular imaging and related areas.

Gang Ho Lee, PhD
February 2013

About the authors

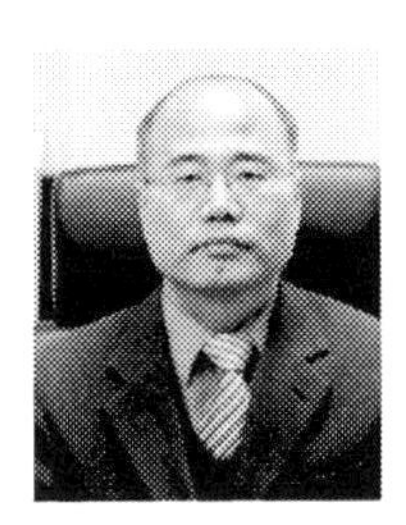

Gang Ho Lee was born in 1961 in South Korea. He received his BSc in chemistry from Korea University, Seoul, South Korea in 1984, his MA in 1988 and his PhD in 1990 in Experimental Physical Chemistry from Johns Hopkins University, Baltimore, USA. He moved to Columbia University, New York, USA as a post-doctoral fellow. He then moved to Riken in Japan as a Science and Technology Agency (STA) fellow. He started an Assistant Professorship in Chemistry at Kyungpook National University (KNU), Taegu, South Korea in 1993. He is currently a full Professor at Chemistry Department and also a joint Professor at the Nanoscience and Nanotechnology Department at KNU. His current research interest covers the synthesis and characterization of surface modified nanoparticles for biomedical applications.

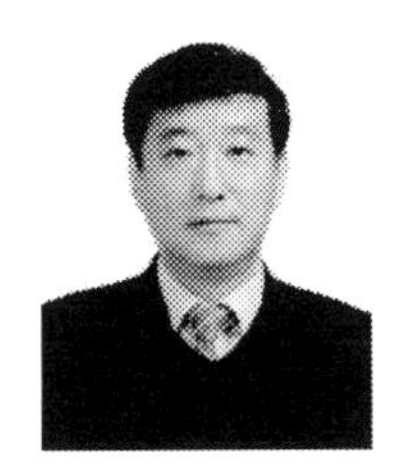

Yongmin Chang received his PhD in Physics from the University of Notre Dame in 1994. Following his PhD, he moved to the University of Illinois at Urbana-Champaign as a post-doc, where he focused on the development and evaluation of lanthanide compounds as MRI contrast agent. He began his faculty appointment as Assistant Professor in

Radiology at Kyungpook National University, College of Medicine in 1997. He became Associate Professor in 2001 and Professor in 2005. Currently, he has a joint faculty appointment in the Molecular Medicine, Biomedical Engineering and Nanoscience Department at Kyungpook National University.

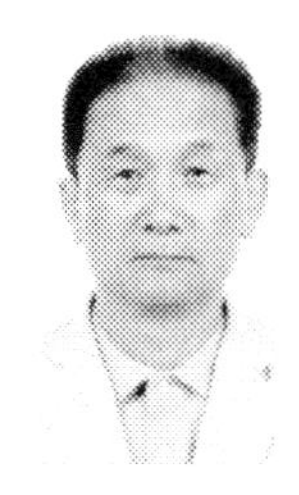

Tae-Jeong Kim received his BSc and MS in Chemistry from Korea University in 1976 and 1978, respectively, and his PhD in Inorganic Chemistry from the University of British Columbia in 1984 under the supervision of Professor W. R. Cullen. He then joined Doctor R. H. Fish in the Lawrence Berkeley Laboratory as a post-doctoral fellow. After spending one year there he began his independent career at Kyungpook National University in 1986, where he now holds a full professorship. His current research interests are Materials and Medicinal Inorganic Chemistry.

1

Introduction to biomedical imaging

DOI: 10.1533/9780081000663.1

Abstract: This chapter defines biomedical imaging and briefly introduces various imaging modalities and imaging agents. These include magnetic resonance imaging (MRI), X-ray computed tomography (CT), ultrasound imaging (USI), positron emission tomography (PET), single photon emission computed tomography (SPECT), fluorescent imaging (FI), and corresponding imaging agents.

Key words: biomedical imaging, MRI, CT, USI, PET, SPECT, FI, imaging agents.

1.1 What is biomedical imaging?

Biomedical imaging is an area that visually characterizes living objects *in vitro* and *in vivo* such as cells, tissues, and organs in the human body through various spectroscopic techniques. Functional, biological, and metabolic processes can also be investigated. Nowadays biomedical imaging is an essential tool to diagnose and treat diseases such as cancer, and a variety of biomedical imaging modalities are now available. These include magnetic resonance imaging (MRI),

X-ray computed tomography (CT), ultrasound imaging (USI), positron emission tomography (PET), single photon emission computed tomography (SPECT), and fluorescent imaging (FI). The operation of biomedical imaging critically depends on the imaging agent. In MRI, CT, and USI, images are improved with an imaging agent through contrast enhancement. In PET, SPECT, and FI, imaging agents are essential components in obtaining clear images.

Biomedical imaging rapidly developed in both imaging tools and imaging agents. As a result, both resolution and sensitivity have been improved. In addition, multi-imaging modalities, such as MRI-CT and MRI-PET, are now being developed. They can provide us with complementary information and some of them are already available in the market. Sensitivity is further improved by integration of a targeting molecule into the imaging agent. A drug can be conjugated to an imaging agent for both diagnosis and treatment (so-called theragnosis) of diseases such as cancer.

1.2 Various imaging modalities now available

It is worth briefly introducing some imaging modalities and imaging agents that are now available. Ultrasmall lanthanide oxide nanoparticles can be used in various imaging modalities, including MRI, CT, USI, PET, SPECT, and FI. USI costs are low and so is the most frequently used to check health and diagnose disease. CT and MRI are more expensive than USI and so are less frequently used. PET and SPECT are the most expensive and least frequently used, mainly due to radio-isotopes being used as imaging agents. FI is very sensitive but mostly used for research purposes owing to its imaging depth limits. Each one of these imaging techniques is described below.

1.2.1 Ultrasound imaging (USI)

Ultrasound imaging is a truly non-invasive imaging modality because it makes use of non-ionizing ultrasonic radiation [1]. Therefore, it does not harm the human body. The frequency in USI ranges from 2 to 18 MHz. The ultrasound wave is generated by a piezoelectric transducer (PZT) and travels through the body, where it can be focused to the desired depth for imaging. The returning ultrasound wave (i.e. the echo) to the tranducer is transformed into an electrical signal and finally into an image.

The ultrasound image can be improved by using contrast agents through echo signal enhancement [2,3]. The currently used USI contrast agents are microbubbles, which contain air or a specific gas such as nitrogen and perfluorocarbon in a lipid, galactose, polymer, or albumin shell. These microbubbles range from 1 to 5 μm in diameter. A USI contrast agent is intravenously injected into the body. When an ultrasound wave passes through a microbubble, the gas inside that microbubble compresses and oscillates, reflecting the ultrasound wave and thus enhancing the echo signal. The echo signal can be further enhanced if the ultrasound wave resonates inside the microbubble. Under such conditions, even a small blood vessel can be imaged. If a USI contrast agent is conjugated with a targeting molecule, such as an antibody or a peptide, the echo signal from the targeted region can be further boosted. A USI contrast agent can also be applied to theragnosis if a drug is conjugated with it. Some commercial USI contrast agents are listed in Table 1.1.

Table 1.1 Some of the USI contrast agents in the market

Trade name	Company	Microbubble structure	
		Shell	Gas
Optison™	GE Healthcare, USA	albumin	octafluoropropane
Levovist®	Scherring, Germany	lipid/galatose	air
Definity®	Lantheus Medical Imaging, Inc., USA	lipid	octafluoropropane
Albunex®	MBI, USA and Nycomed Imaging AS, Norway	albumin	air

1.2.2 X-ray imaging and X-ray computed tomography (CT)

X-ray imaging is frequently used to check for the presence of disease during health examinations and is widely used to image bone structure. The energy of X-rays is so high that it corresponds to ionizing radiation. Therefore it is harmful to the human body if exposed to it for a long time and so cannot be considered a truly non-invasive imaging modality. It may damage DNA and so long-time exposure to X-rays should be avoided, especially for infants.

Wilhelm Röntgen discovered the X-ray and first applied it to bone imaging. The image is obtained by targeting a short pulse of hard X-rays (5–100 keV) to a specific part of the body and detecting the outgoing X-ray beam through the body. The image is then produced on a two-dimensional (2-D) photographic film. Thus, X-ray imaging is based on the reduction of the beam as it passes through the body, so the difference in attenuation of the X-ray beam between organs, tissues, and bones produces the contrast and thus an image. As the X-ray is nearly transparent for soft tissues, X-ray imaging is useful for bones and hardened parts such as diseased areas in tissues.

X-ray computed tomography (CT) is a 2-D image made up of slices that are obtained as both the X-ray beam and detector rotate around the body. After a complete rotation, a slice image is constructed with the help of a sophisticated computation using a computer. The X-ray beam and detector are moved along the body axis and another image slice is obtained from this further scan. A 3-dimensional (3-D) image can be constructed from a continuous set of 2-D image slices. Its spatial resolution and sensitivity are comparable to that of MRI.

X-ray and CT images can be improved using a contrast agent, which strongly attenuates the X-ray beam intensity reaching the detector. Therefore, even soft tissues and tiny blood vessels can be imaged at a high resolution. Two types (i.e. oral and intravascular) of contrast agents are in the market (Table 1.2). The intravascular contrast agents are mostly tri-iodinated organic compounds with hydrophilic functional groups for water-solubility [4,5]. The oral contrast agents are mainly used for imaging stomach and intestines. Improved images can be obtained if a contrast agent is

Table 1.2 **Some of the X-ray (or CT) contrast agents in the market**

Brand name	Chemical	Company	Usage
–	$BaSO_4$	–	Digestive system
Omnipaque™	$C_{19}H_{26}I_3N_3O_9$	GE Healthcare, USA	Intravascular
Visipaque™	$C_{35}H_{44}I_6N_6O_{15}$	GE Healthcare, USA	Intravascular
Ultravist®	$C_{18}H_{24}I_3N_3O_8$	Bayer Healthcare, Germany	Intravascular
Isovue®	$C_{17}H_{22}I_3N_3O_3$	Bracco, New Zealand	Intravascular

conjugated with a targeting molecule such as an antibody or peptide. On the other hand, gold nanoparticles can provide an enhanced contrast superior to an iodine contrast agent, because gold has an X-ray attenuation power of ~2.7 times that of iodine [6]. Therefore, even the tiniest of blood vessels can be imaged with gold nanoparticles.

1.2.3 Magnetic resonance imaging (MRI)

Magnetic resonance imaging (MRI) makes use of nuclear magnetic resonance (NMR) of protons in the body to produce images [7]. It is a truly non-invasive imaging technique, because radiofrequency is used as the radiation source. Due to an ample existence of protons in the body in the form of water, proteins, fats, etc., signal intensity and spatial resolution is better than with USI and comparable to CT. MRI is very useful for imaging soft tissues such as brain, muscles, heart, and so on. Local protons have different densities and relaxation rates, from which images are obtained from differences in contrast. A normal tissue can be differentiated from a cancerous tissue because of their different proton densities and relaxation rates related to angiogenesis.

MRI contrast agents help to improve images through contrast enhancement. There are two types of MRI contrast agents based on proton relaxation mechanisms: T_1 and T_2 MRI contrast agents. The former is called a positive contrast agent because it makes the contrast brighter [8,9], whereas the latter is called a negative contrast agent because it makes the contrast darker [10]. The dextran coated superparamagnetic iron oxide (SPIO) nanoparticle is a well-known T_2 MRI contrast agent. On the other hand, T_1 MRI contrast agents are mostly Gd(III)-chelates. The latter prevail in the market nowadays. The former is usually limited to the liver because it is accumulated into the liver due to its large particle size. Some of clinically used MRI contrast agents are listed in Table 1.3.

1.2.4 Positron emission tomography (PET)

Positron emission tomography (PET) is a chemical-based imaging modality [11]. It makes use of a radionuclide that emits a positron (i.e. an electron with a positive charge). The radionuclides used in PET include ^{11}C (half life, $t_{1/2}$ = ~20 min), ^{13}N (half life, $t_{1/2}$ = ~10 min), ^{15}O (half life, $t_{1/2}$ = ~2 min), ^{18}F (half life, $t_{1/2}$ = ~110 min), and ^{82}Rb (half life, $t_{1/2}$ = ~1.27 min), all of which have short half-lives [12,13]. A radionuclide is typically incorporated into glucose or a glucose analog or other compound.

A PET agent is injected intravenously into the body. The most commonly used PET agent is fluorodeoxyglucose (FDG) because of a relatively long half-life of ^{18}F compared to other radionuclides. After injection, the agent circulates through the blood vessel and then accumulates in the region

Table 1.3 Some of the MRI contrast agents in the market

Brand name	Chemical	Company	Usage	
Magnevist®	$[Gd(DTPA)(H_2O)]^{2-}$	Scherring, Germany	T_1	Intravascular
Dotarem®	$[Gd(DOTA)(H_2O)]^-$	Guerbet, France	T_1	Intravascular
Omniscan™	$[Gd(DTPA\text{-}BMA)(H_2O)]$	GE Healthcare, USA	T_1	Intravascular
Gadovist®	$[Gd(DO3A\text{-}butrol)(H_2O)]$	Scherring, Germany	T_1	Intravascular
Resovist®	$Fe_3O_4/\gamma\text{-}Fe_2O_3$@ carboxydextran	Scherring, Germany	T_2	Intravascular
Lumirem®	SPIO	Advanced Magnetics, USA	T_2	Oral

of interest. An emitted positron from the radionuclide travels through the body for a short distance of ~1 mm and then the positron decelerates due to kinetic energy loss when interacting with an electron (i.e. the so-called positron-electron annihilation), from which a γ-ray is generated. The PET system detects the γ-ray using a scintillation detector. The PET image provides us with an exact location of diseases such as cancer. In addition, the metabolic processes of organs in the body can be investigated.

Chemicals used in PET are generally manufactured at a hospital because of the short half-lives of the radionuclides [12,13]. The radionuclides are generally produced using a cyclotron that is installed near to the PET imager at the hospital.

1.2.5 Single photon emission computed tomography (SPECT)

Single photon emission computed tomography (SPECT) is a chemical-based nuclear imaging modality similar to PET [13]. However, by using a gamma camera, SPECT directly detects the γ-ray that is emitted from a radionuclide such as ^{99m}Tc (half life, $t_{1/2}$=~6 h), ^{123}I (half life, $t_{1/2}$=~13 h), ^{131}I (half life, $t_{1/2}$=~20 min), or ^{111}Ir (half life, $t_{1/2}$=~67 h), in all compound forms. A SPECT agent is intravenously injected into the body. The resolution of SPECT (=~1 cm) is much lower than that of PET because of the much longer half-life of the radionuclide compared to that of the PET agent.

The chemicals are sold by pharmaceuticals (Table 1.4), because the long half-lives of the radionuclides means that they can be shipped to the hospital [13,14]. Since SPECT agents are mostly removed from the body through urine, the bladder should be voided as soon as possible to minimize the radiation dose after the intravenous injection.

Table 1.4 Some of the SPECT agents in the market

Brand name	Chemical	Company	Usage
Myoview™	^{99m}Tc-tetrofosmin (= [1,2-bis[di-(2-ethoxyethyl) phosphino]ethane]$_2$)	GE Healthcare, USA	Cardiac Imaging, Intravascular
Cardiolite®	^{99m}Tc-sestamibi (= [methoxyisobutylisonitrile]$_6$)	Lantheus Medical Imaging, USA	Cardiac Imaging, Intravascular
Ceretec™	^{99m}Tc-HMPAO (= hexamethylpropyleneamine oxime)	GE Healthcare, USA	Brain, Intravascular

1.2.6 Fluorescent imaging (FI)

Fluorescent imaging (FI) is a chemical-based imaging modality, which makes use of light ranging from the visible to near infrared (NIR) as an excitation source and thus is a non-invasive imaging modality. Its sensitivity and resolution are very high [15–18]. The FI is extremely useful in locating disease due to its high sensitivity and high resolution, which are only limited by the optical device. However, a severe disadvantage of FI over the other imaging modalities already described is a limited imaging depth owing to absorption and scattering of light by biological objects, making clinical applications difficult. In the visible region, the penetration depth of light is a few millimeters. In the NIR region, the penetration depth can be increased by up to a few centimeters. Therefore, the FI is not common in clinical use and has been mainly applied to cell and small animal imaging in research.

FI entirely depends on the imaging agent. The fluorescent imaging agents should be highly water-soluble, biocompatible, photostable, and intensely fluorescent. Until now, organic dyes have been commonly used as fluorescent imaging agents [15]. They have very strong fluorescent intensities but develop photobleaching and photodecomposition after multiple uses (i.e. poor photostability) and wide emission bandwidths due to widespread transition energy levels, making multiplex imaging difficult.

Quantum dots (QDs) can be also used as FI agents. They provide high fluorescent intensity like a dye but have a narrow bandwidth and a high photostability, which is superior to a dye [16]. Their wavelength is tunable from the visible to infrared by varying particle diameter or composition. However, one shortcoming of the QD is its inherent toxicity [19], making clinical applications undesirable.

Lanthanide elements in the form of complex or oxide nanoparticle are potential FI agents. Lanthanide oxide nanoparticles show fluorescent properties similar to those of QDs, except for weaker fluorescent intensity [17,18]. Some of them are nearly non-toxic, which is of great advantage in clinical applications. Their emission wavelength depends on Ln(III) ions, spanning from the visible to infrared. The up-converting nano-systems composed of mixed lanthanide oxide nanoparticles, in which one of Ln(III) ions is a near infrared absorber and the other is a visible emitter, can provide an increased imaging depth of up to a few centimeters. Furthermore, the fluorescent intensity of lanthanide oxide nanoparticles increases with decreasing particle diameter [20,21], which is beneficial in clinical applications because only ultrasmall nanoparticles can be excreted from the body through the renal system [22].

1.3 References

1. Wells, P.T. (2006), 'Ultrasound imaging', *Phys. Med. Biol.*, 51: R83–R98.
2. Calliada, F., Campani, R., Bottinelli, O., Bozzini, A. and Sommaruga, M.G. (1998), 'Ultrasound contrast agents: basic principles', *Eur. J. Radiol.*, 27: S157–S160.
3. Stride, E. and Saffari, N. (2003), 'Microbubble ultrasound contrast agents: a review', *Proc. Instn. Mech. Engrs.* (part H: *J. Eng. Med.*), 217: 429–47.
4. Lusic, H. and Grinstaff, M.W. (2013), 'X-ray-computed tomography contrast agents', *Chem. Rev.*, 113: 1641–66.
5. Yu, S.-B. and Watson, A.D. (1999), 'Metal-based X-ray contrast media', *Chem. Rev.*, 99: 2353–78.

6. Hainfeld, J.F., Slatkin, D.N., Focella, T.M. and Smilowitz, H.M. (2006), 'Gold nanoparticles: a new X-ray contrast agent', *British J. Radiol.*, 79: 248–53.
7. Hashemi, R.H., Bradley, W.G. and Lisanti, C.J. (2004), *MRI The Basics*, 2nd edn, New York: Lippincott Williams & Wilkins.
8. Lauffer, R.B. (1987), 'Paramagnetic metal complexes as water proton relaxation agents for NMR imaging: theory and design', *Chem. Rev.*, 87: 901–27.
9. Caravan, P., Ellison, J.J., McMurry, T.J. and Lauffer, R.B. (1999), 'Gadolinium(III) chelates as MRI contrast agents: structure, dynamics, and applications', *Chem. Rev.*, 99: 2293–52.
10. Reimer, P. and Balzer, T. (2003), 'Ferucarbotran (Resovist): a new clinically approved RES-specific contrast agent for contrast-enhanced MRI of the liver: properties, clinical development, and applications', *Eur. Radiol.*, 13: 1266–76.
11. Bailey, D.L., Townsend, D.W., Valk, P.E. and Maisey, M.W. (2005), *Positron Emission Tomography: Basic Sciences*, New Jersey: Springer-Verlag.
12. Anderson, C.J. and Welch, M.J. (1999), 'Radiometal-labeled agents (non-technetium) for diagnostic imaging', *Chem. Rev.*, 99: 2219–34.
13. Wadas, T.J., Wong, E.H., Weisman, G.R. and Anderson, C.J. (2010), 'Coordinating radiometals of copper, gallium, indium, yttrium, and zirconium for PET and SPECT imaging of disease', *Chem. Rev.*, 110: 2858–902.
14. Liu, S. and Edwards, D.S. (1999), '^{99}Tc-labeled small peptides as diagnostic radiopharmaceuticals', *Chem. Rev.*, 99: 2235–68.
15. Kovar, J.L., Simpson, M.A., Schutz-Geschwender, A. and Olive, D.M. (2007), 'A systematic approach to the

development of fluorescent contrast agents for optical imaging of mouse cancer models', *Anal. Biochem.*, 367: 1–12.

16. Michalet, X., Pinaud, F.F., Bentolila, L.A., Tsay, J.M., Doose, S. et al. (2005), 'Quantum dots for live cells, *in vivo* imaging, and diagnostics', *Science*, 307: 538–44.
17. Bünzli, J.-C.G. (2010), 'Lanthanide luminescence for biomedical analyses and imaging', *Chem. Rev.*, 110: 2729–55.
18. Eliseeva, S.V. and Bünzli, J.-C.G. (2010), 'Lanthanide luminescence for functional materials and bio-sciences', *Chem. Soc. Rev.*, 39: 1–380.
19. Hardman, R. (2006), 'A toxicologic review of quantum dots: toxicity depends on physicochemical and environmental factors', *Environ. Health Perpect.*, 114: 165–72.
20. Wakefield, G., Keron, H.A., Dobson, P.J. and Hutchison, J.L. (1999), 'Synthesis and properties of sub-50-nm europium oxide nanoparticles', *J. Colloid Interface Sci.*, 215: 179–82.
21. Goldburt, E.T., Kulkarni, B., Bhargava, R.N., Taylor, J. and Libera, M. (1997), 'Size dependent efficiency in Tb doped Y_2O_3 nanocrystalline phosphor', *J. Lumin.*, 72–4: 190–2.
22. Choi, H.S., Liu, W., Misra, P., Tanaka, E., Zimmer, J.P. et al. (2007), 'Renal clearance of quantum dots', *Nat. Biotechnology*, 25: 1165–70.

2

Properties and possible application areas

DOI: 10.1533/9780081000694.15

Abstract: This chapter briefly discusses the physical and chemical properties of ultrasmall lanthanide oxide nanoparticles and their possible application to biomedical imagings such as MRI, CT, FI, and multimodal imaging and thermal neutron capture therapy (NCT).

Key words: ultrasmall lanthanide oxide nanoparticle, properties, application area.

2.1 Introduction

Ultrasmall lanthanide oxide nanoparticles can be applied to a variety of imaging areas as imaging agents by using their magnetic, optical, and X-ray attenuation properties. These nanoparticles can also be used as therapeutic agents by using the thermal neutron capturing property of ^{157}Gd. This chapter discusses their physical properties and areas of application.

2.1.1 Magnetic properties

The magnetic properties of ultrasmall lanthanide oxide nanoparticles arise from 4f-electrons of Ln(III) (Table 2.1) [1]. Both bulk and lanthanide oxide nanoparticles have been known to be paramagnetic from room temperature to a few kelvins. Therefore, the magnetic moment of a lanthanide oxide nanoparticle is nearly the sum of those of individual Ln(III) ions in a lanthanide oxide nanoparticle. However, paramagnetic, ultrasmall lanthanide oxide nanoparticles show appreciable magnetic moments at room temperature, which can be used for MRI contrast agents. As shown in Figure 2.1, D-glucuronic acid coated ultrasmall holmium oxide nanoparticles in an aqueous solution can be drawn by a magnet, owing to their appreciable magnetic moment at room temperature.

Due to a strong spin-orbit coupling of 4f-electrons with a spin-orbit coupling constant of ~1000 cm^{-1} [2], only the

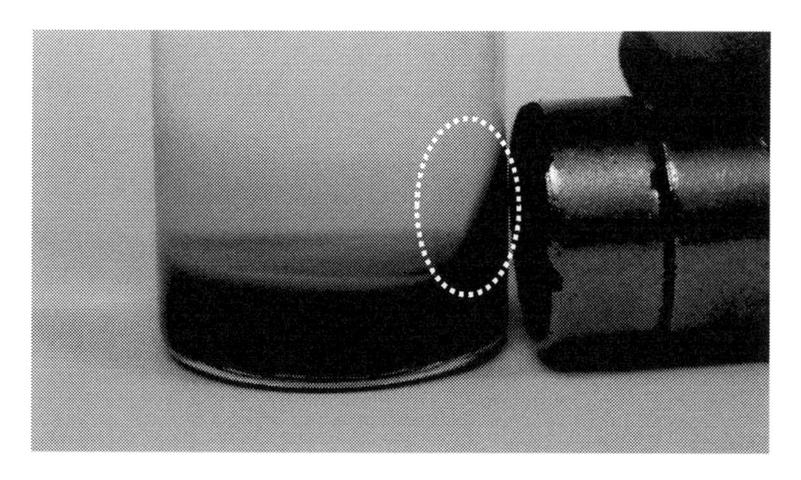

Figure 2.1 D-glucuronic acid coated holmium oxide nanoparticles in an aqueous solution drawn by a magnet (indicated with a dotted circle)

ground J-state is populated, except for an Eu(III) that has a temperature-dependent population of low-lying excited J-states. In fact, magnetic moments of Ln(III) theoretically calculated using a Landé formula [3] with this ground J-state population are consistent with those observed, except for Eu(III) (Table 2.1).

The 4f-electrons are compacted close to the nucleus and so are generally unaffected by ligands, whereas diffuse 3d-electrons are largely affected by ligands. In fact, a ligand field splitting of Ln(III) ions is only ~100 cm^{-1}, whereas that of 3d-transition metal ions is ~20 000 cm^{-1} [4]. Therefore, the ligand effect on magnetic properties of Ln(III) and thus on ultrasmall lanthanide oxide nanoparticles is minor. This also applies to optical properties of ultrasmall lanthanide oxide nanoparticles. Therefore, surface Ln(III) in a ultrasmall lanthanide oxide nanoparticle will significantly contribute to both water proton relaxation and fluorescent intensity. It has been found that r_1 of gadolinium oxide nanoparticles is optimal at particle diameter (d) of 1 to 2.5 nm [5]. It has also been found that a fluorescent intensity of europium oxide

Table 2.1 Magnetic and optical properties of some selected lanthanide (Ln) ions useful for biomedical imaging [1]

Ln(III)	Ground State configuration	Number of unpaired 4f electrons	Color	Theoretical magnetic moment (μB)	Observed magnetic moment (μB)
Eu(III)	$^7F_0$	6 ($4f^6$)	pink	0	3.3–3.5
Gd(III)	$^8S_{7/2}$	7 ($4f^7$)	–	7.94	7.9–8.0
Tb(III)	$^7F_6$	6 ($4f^8$)	green	9.72	9.5–9.8
Dy(III)	$^6H_{15/2}$	5 ($4f^9$)	–	10.65	10.4–10.6
Ho(III)	$^5I_8$	4 ($4f^{10}$)	–	10.6	10.4–10.7
Er(III)	$^4I_{15/2}$	3 ($4f^{11}$)	–	9.58	9.4–9.6

nanoparticles increases with decreasing d [6,7]. As listed in Table 2.1, all of Ln(III) ions, except for Eu(III), possess large magnetic moments. Therefore, their ultrasmall oxide nanoparticles could be useful as MRI contrast agents.

MRI is based on proton relaxation; the proton relaxes in two ways. One is longitudinal (T_1) relaxation and the other is transverse (T_2) relaxation [8]. For surface coated nanoparticles, an outer sphere model can be applied to T_1 relaxation, because water protons are indirectly in contact with Ln(III) in a nanoparticle due to the ligand [9]. The T_1 relaxation of the proton is accelerated by an electron spin magnetic moment. Therefore, the longitudinal water proton relaxivity (r_1) will be proportional to the square of the spin magnetic moment (m_s) of a Ln(III) ion times number (N) of Ln(III) ions in a nanoparticle contributing to T_1 relaxation (mostly those close to the proton). Thus:

$$r_1 \propto N m_s^2 \quad [2.1]$$

Only Gd(III) in Table 2.1 possesses spins of $S = 7/2$ with no orbital magnetic moment component (i.e. $L = 0$). Therefore, r_1 of ultrasmall gadolinium oxide nanoparticles will be large. Large r_1 values that are several times larger than those of Gd(III)-chelates [9] have been observed only in ultrasmall gadolinium oxide nanoparticles, whereas other lanthanide oxide nanoparticles showed negligible r_1 values close to zero [10].

However, the T_2 relaxation of a water proton is induced by fluctuations of local magnetic fields generated by nanoparticles [9]. Thus, r_2 value will be proportional to the square of the total magnetic moment (M_{NP}) of a nanoparticle, that is:

$$r_2 \propto M_{NP}^2 \quad [2.2]$$

As shown in Table 2.1, both Dy(III) and Ho(III) ions possess the largest magnetic moment among Ln(III). Therefore, it is expected that their oxide nanoparticles will show large magnetic moments, which has been confirmed by experiment [10]. Their magnetic moment at room temperature will further increase with increasing applied fields, because their magnetic moments are not saturated at room temperature. In fact, the r_2 value of dysprosium oxide nanoparticles was found to be even larger than that of superparamagnetic iron oxide (SPIO) nanoparticles at high applied fields [11,12]. Therefore, both ultrasmall dysprosium oxide and holmium oxide nanoparticles are potential T_2 MRI contrast agents at high MR fields.

Other Ln(III), such as Gd(III), Tb(III), and Er(III), also possess decent magnetic moments at room temperature and thus will be potential T_2 MRI contrast agents at high MR fields. In addition to r_1 and r_2 values, the r_2/r_1 ratio, which is theoretically always greater than one [8], is another important factor in T_1 MRI contrast agents. It should be close to one for T_1 MRI contrast agents, whereas it should be larger for a T_2 MRI contrast agent. Ultrasmall gadolinium oxide nanoparticles satisfy the former condition, whereas other ultrasmall lanthanide oxide nanoparticles satisfy the latter condition [10].

2.1.2 Optical (or fluorescent) properties

Ultrasmall lanthanide oxide nanoparticles have a variety of optical properties owing to 4f-electrons of Ln(III), like magnetic properties [13,14]. Although weaker in fluorescent intensity than dyes and QDs, some lanthanide ions emit appreciable photons in the visible and near infrared regions. The most used Ln(III) ions in the visible region are Eu(III), which emit photons in the red region (615 nm) and Tb(III), which emit photons in the green region (540 nm). Their emission intensities are relatively stronger than the other

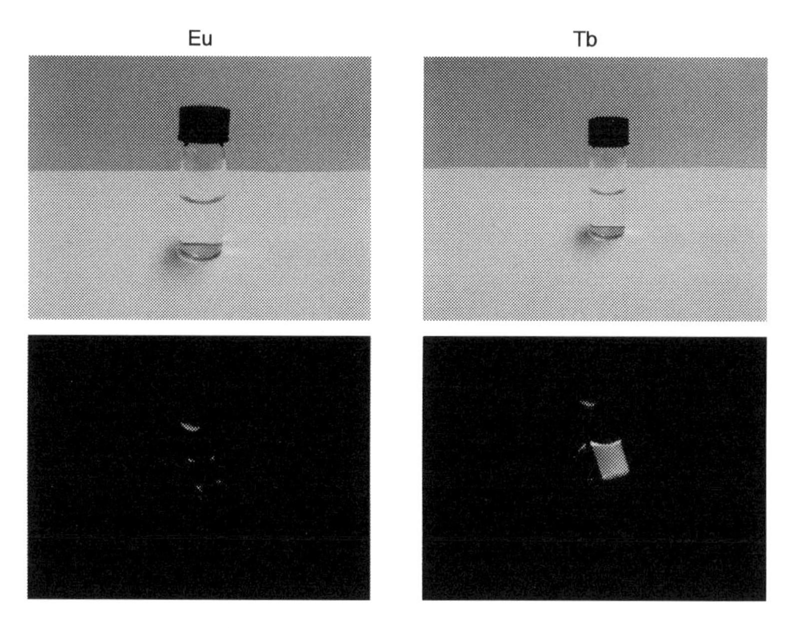

Figure 2.2 Fluorescent Eu(III) (left) and Tb(III) (right) solutions in ethanol after 325 nm UV irradiation: before (top) and after (bottom) UV irradiation

Ln(III) ions given in Table 2.1. Their fluorescent ethanol solutions after 325 nm UV irradiation are shown in Figure 2.2, displaying their red and green emission colors, respectively.

The fluorescent intensity of lanthanide oxide nanoparticles can be maximized by decreasing particle diameters, resulting from reduced excitation migration to quenching sites that are proportional to particle diameters [6,7]. Therefore, the fluorescent imaging is optimal at ultrasmall particle diameters. In addition, after intravenous injection, the ultrasmall nanoparticles can be easily excreted from the body through the renal system, which is a prerequisite for clinical applications, whereas large nanoparticles accumulate in the liver [15].

The fluorescent imaging agents in the visible region have an imaging depth limit of a few millimeters. This can be overcome by using up-converting nano-systems in which one of the Ln(III) ions is a near infrared absorber and the other is a visible emitter [16]. The up-converting nano-systems can provide an increased depth limit of up to a few centimeters. The most commonly used example is an Er(III)/Yb(III) combination, in which Er(III) functions as a visible emitter (540 nm (green) and 654 nm (red)) and Yb(III), as a photosensitizer (i.e. near infrared absorber).

2.1.3 X-ray attenuation property

Lanthanide elements have large X-ray attenuation coefficients [17] for hard X-rays (5–100 keV). This property is useful for X-ray and CT contrast agents. The X-ray attenuation coefficient (μ) or X-ray mass attenuation coefficient (μ/ρ) can be determined from [17]

$$\mu/\rho = x^{-1} \ln(I_0/I) \qquad [2.3]$$

in which ρ is the density (g/cm^3) of the object, x is the mass thickness (g/cm^2) that is obtained from $x = \rho t$, t is the the thickness (cm) of the object, I_0 is the incident X-ray beam intensity, and I is the outcoming X-ray beam intensity. μ or μ/ρ can be obtained by passing a monochromatic X-ray beam and measuring I_0/I (Figure 2.3).

X-ray attenuation coefficients of some selected elements with high μ/ρ values that are useful as X-ray and CT contrast agents are plotted as a function of X-ray photon energy in Figure 2.4 [17]. Gold (Au) has the highest X-ray attenuation coefficient among the elements. The next is tungsten (W), and the third is gadolinium (Gd). However, tri-iodine (I) organic compounds are now clinically used as X-ray and CT contrast agents. As plotted in Figure 2.4, iodine (I) generally

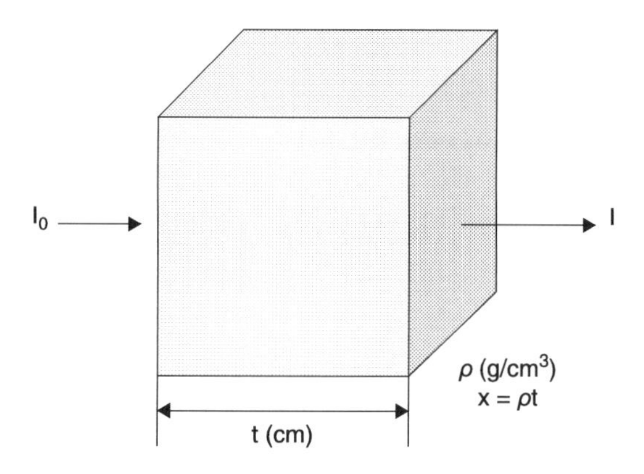

Figure 2.3 A schematic configuration to measure the X-ray attenuation coefficient (μ) or X-ray mass attenuation coefficient (μ/ρ)

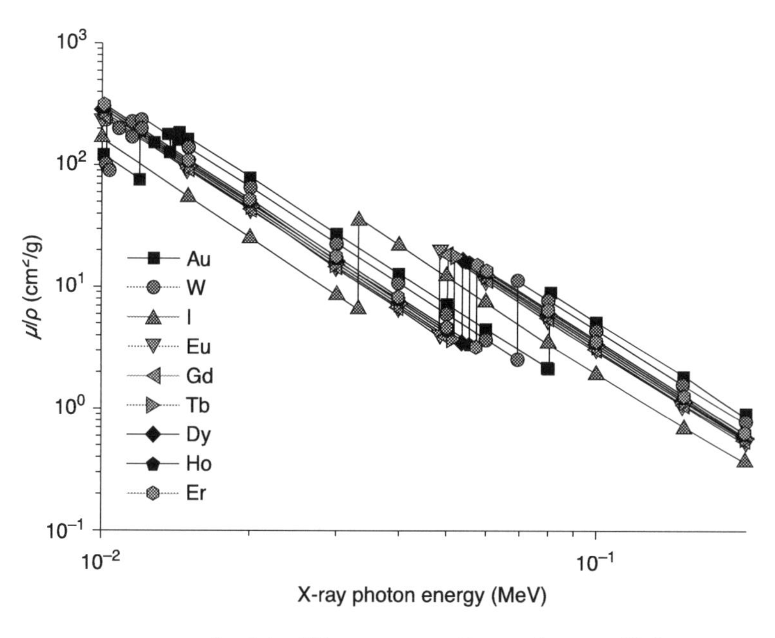

Figure 2.4 A plot of X-ray mass attenuation coefficient (μ/ρ) of some selected elements as a function of X-ray photon energy

has a lower X-ray attenuation coefficient than the other elements. Gd has an X-ray attenuation power that is 2.5 times higher than I. Therefore, ultrasmall gadolinium oxide nanoparticles are potential CT contrast agent. Other lanthanide elements also have X-ray attenuation coefficients higher than I, implying that other ultrasmall lanthanide oxide nanoparticles are also potential X-ray and CT contrast agents. Since ultrasmall lanthanide oxide nanoparticles also have additional imaging functions, such as MRI and FI, they could be used as multimodal imaging agents.

As mentioned in Chapter 1, bones and hardened areas of disease in the body can be imaged with X-rays, because an X-ray beam is nearly transparent for soft tissues and blood vessels. However, soft tissues and blood vessels can be imaged with X-ray and CT contrast agents in high resolution.

2.1.4 Thermal neutron capture cross-section

Gadolinium (^{157}Gd, natural abundance = 15.7%) has a high thermal neutron capture cross-section of 257 000 barns (1 barn = 10^{-24} m^2, the size of the uranium nucleus) [18]. This corresponds to the largest value among the known stable isotopes. Here, the thermal neutron has energy of less than 0.1 eV. ^{157}Gd has a ~67 times higher thermal neutron capture cross-section than ^{10}B (natural abundance = 19.6%) with 3840 barns, which has been used for boron neutron capture therapy (BNCT).

Neutron capture therapy (NCT) was begun with ^{10}B. BNCT was first suggested by G.L. Locher at the Franklin Institute in Pennsylvania, USA. After this, many researchers had begun using BNCT in USA, Europe, Asia, etc. NCT generally depends on thermal neutron capture cross-section of capturing atoms and nuclear reaction products. ^{10}B becomes excited into ^{11}B after capturing a thermal neutron, which then generates a ^{7}Li and α-particle (Equation 2.4). Both ^{7}Li and α-particles can contribute to cancer cell damage by denaturing the double-helix of the DNA in the cancer cell nucleus. Both ^{7}Li and α-particles have a penetration depth of less than 10 μm, corresponding to the diameter of a cell. Therefore, ^{10}B-chemicals should be close to or inside the cancer cell nucleus for effective DNA damage:

$$^{10}B + n_{thermal} \rightarrow [^{11}B] \rightarrow \alpha\ (1.47\,MeV) + {}^{7}Li\ (0.84\,MeV) \quad [2.4]$$

$$^{157}Gd + n_{thermal} \rightarrow {}^{158}Gd + \gamma(7.88\,MeV) + ACK - electrons\ (4.2\,keV) \quad [2.5]$$

^{157}Gd captures a thermal neutron and becomes ^{158}Gd, which then generates γ-ray and electrons (Equation 2.5). Among the reaction products, Auger and Coster-Kronig (ACK) electrons mainly participate in cancer cell damage by indirectly damaging DNA in the cancer cell nucleus. ACK electrons react with water and then generate reactive OH^-, which denatures the double-helix DNA, thus damaging the cancer cell. Since ACK electrons have a short penetration distance of less than 10 μm, corresponding to a cell diameter, ^{157}Gd-chemicals should be close to or inside the cancer cell nucleus, like in the case of BNCT. The high energy γ-ray is also effective in breaking up cancer cells. A theoretical simulation study showed that a 5 Gy (1 gray = 1 J/kg) is enough to damage cancer cells [19]. However, ACK electrons are more useful than high energy γ-rays, because ACK electrons can damage only cancer cells if they are targeted to those cells, whereas high energy γ-ray can also damage normal cells because of its long penetration depth (10 cm).

The success of NCT critically depends on targeting of the chemicals to the cancer cells and causing no damage to normal cells. NCT will be extremely useful for a variety of cancers, especially for those that cannot be treated by conventional surgery. These include malignant brain cancer, hematologic malignancy, and metastatic cancer.

2.2 Possible application areas

Ultrasmall lanthanide oxide nanoparticles can be applied to a variety of biomedical imaging and NCT, using their properties as described above. Their areas of application are summarized in Table 2.2.

It is worth mentioning that ultrasmall lanthanide oxide nanoparticles should be non-toxic for biomedical applications. Therefore, they should be surface modified with hydrophilic biocompatible ligands for non-toxicity and water-solubility. Their particle diameters should be as small as possible to allow for renal excretion through the kidneys because they cannot be digested inside the body through normal metabolic processes. It is known that nanoparticles can be excreted

Table 2.2 Possible application areas of ultrasmall lanthanide oxide nanoparticles

Nanoparticle	Possible application area
Eu_2O_3	FI, CT
Gd_2O_3	T_1 MRI, CT, NCT (^{157}Gd)
Tb_2O_3	T_2 MRI, FI, CT
Dy_2O_3	T_2 MRI, CT
Ho_2O_3	T_2 MRI, CT
Er_2O_3	T_2 MRI, CT

effectively from the body through the renal system when the particle diameter is less than 3 nm [15].

2.3 References

1. Greenwood, N.N. and Earnshaw, A. (1997), *Chemistry of the Elements*, 2nd edn, Oxford, UK: Butterworth-Heinemann, p. 1243.
2. Carlin, R.L. (1986), *Magnetochemistry*, Berlin: Springer-Verlag, p. 238.
3. Cullity, B.D. (1972), *Introduction to Magnetic Materials*, Reading, UK: Addison-Wesley Publishing Company, p. 102.
4. Cotton, F.A. and Wilkinson, G. (1980), *Advanced Inorganic Chemistry*, 4th edn, New York: Wiley-Interscience, p. 646 and 984.
5. Park, J.Y., Baek, M.J., Choi, E.S., Woo, S., Kim, J.H. et al. (2009), 'Paramagnetic ultrasmall gadolinium oxide nanoparticles as advanced T_1 MRI contrast agent: account for large longitudinal relaxivity, optimal particle diameter, and *in vivo* T_1 MR images', *ACS Nano*, 3: 3663–9.
6. Wakefield, G., Keron, H.A., Dobson, P.J. and Hutchison, J.L. (1999), 'Synthesis and properties of sub-50-nm europium oxide nanoparticles', *J. Colloid Interface Sci.*, 215: 179–82.
7. Goldburt, E.T., Kulkarni, B., Bhargava, R.N., Taylor, J. and Libera, M. (1997), 'Size dependent efficiency in Tb doped Y_2O_3 nanocrystalline phosphor', *J. Lumin.*, 72–4: 190–2.
8. Hashemi, R.H., Bradley, W.G.. and Lisanti, C.J. (2004), *MRI The Basics*, 2nd edn, New York: Lippincott Williams & Wilkins.

9. Lauffer, R.B. (1987), 'Paramagnetic metal complexes as water proton relaxation agents for NMR imaging: theory and design', *Chem. Rev.*, 87: 901–27.
10. Kattel, K., Park, J.Y., Xu, W., Kim, H.G., Lee, E.J. et al. (2011), 'A facile synthesis, *in vitro* and *in vivo* MR studies of D-glucuronic acid-coated ultrasmall Ln_2O_3 (Ln = Eu, Gd, Dy, Ho, and Er) nanoparticles as a new potential MRI contrast agent', *ACS Appl. Mater. Interfaces*, 3: 3325–34.
11. Norek, M., Kampert, E., Zeitler, U. and Peters, J.A. (2008), 'Tuning of the size of Dy_2O_3 nanoparticles for optimal performance as an MRI contrast agent', *J. Am. Chem. Soc.*, 130: 5335–40.
12. Norek, M., Pereira, G.A., Geraldes, C.F.G.C., Denkova, A., Zhou, W. and Peters, J.A. (2007), 'NMR transversal relaxivity of suspensions of lanthanide oxide nanoparticles', *J. Phys. Chem. C*, 111: 10240–6.
13. Bünzli, J.-C.G. (2010), 'Lanthanide luminescence for biomedical analyses and imaging', *Chem. Rev.*, 110: 2729–55.
14. Eliseeva, S.V. and Bünzli, J.-C.G. (2010), 'Lanthanide luminescence for functional materials and bio-sciences', *Chem. Soc. Rev.*, 39: 1–380.
15. Choi, H.S., Liu, W., Misra, P., Tanaka, E., Zimmer, J.P. et al. (2007), 'Renal clearance of quantum dots', *Nat. Biotechnology*, 25: 1165–70.
16. Wang, F., Han, Y., Lim, C.S., Lu, Y., Wang, J. et al. (2010), 'Simultaneous phase and size control of up-conversion nanocrystals through lanthanide doping', *Nature*, 463: 1061–5.
17. Hubbell, J.H. and Seltzer, S.M. (1995), 'Tables of X-ray mass attenuation coefficients and mass energy-absorption coefficients from 1 keV to 20 MeV for elements Z = 1 to 92 and 48 additional substances

of dosimetric interest', NIST Technical Report (PB-95-220539/XAB).

18. Mughabghab, S.F. (2003), 'Thermal neutron capture cross-sections: Resonance integrals and g-factors', IAEA Nuclear Data Section, Wagramer Strasse 5, A-1400, Vienna.
19. Masiakowski, J.T., Horton, J.L and Peters, L.J. (1992), 'Gadolinium neutron capture therapy for brain tumors: a computer study', *Med. Phys.*, 19: 1277–84.

3

Synthesis and surface modification

DOI: 10.1533/9780081000694.29

Abstract: This chapter discusses synthesis and surface modification of ultrasmall lanthanide oxide nanoparticles. A polyol method is typically used to synthesize ultrasmall lanthanide oxide nanoparticles. The surface modification with water-soluble and the biocompatible ligand can be carried out in one-pot synthesis.

Key words: synthesis, polyol method, surface modification, one-pot.

3.1 Synthesis

3.1.1 High temperature polyol method

Although a variety of synthetic methods to produce 3-dimentional (3-d)-transition metal oxide nanoparticles have been reported to date, all of them cannot be applied to synthesize lanthanide (Ln) oxide nanoparticles (chemical formula: Ln_2O_3). For instance, when trivalent lanthanide ions react with hydroxide ions in an aqueous solution, lanthanide hydroxide ($Ln(OH)_3$) nanorods are mainly produced instead of lanthanide oxide nanoparticles due to high dehydration energies from $Ln(OH)_3$ into Ln_2O_3, whereas 3-d-transition metal ions readily form metal oxide nanoparticles due to relatively low dehydration energies [1]. Therefore, lanthanide oxide nanoparticles should be produced at elevated temperatures (180–200 °C) in solvents with high boiling points such as diethylene glycol (DEG) [2] or triethylene glycol (TEG) [3]. The suggested formation mechanism of Ln_2O_3 nanoparticles in a high temperature polyol method is

$$\begin{aligned} &Ln(III) + 3OH^- \rightarrow Ln(OH)_3 \\ &Ln(OH)_3 \rightarrow LnOOH + H_2O \\ &2LnOOH \rightarrow Ln_2O_3 + H_2O \end{aligned} \qquad [3.1]$$

Using a high temperature polyol method, ultrasmall nanoparticles can be synthesized. A subsequent surface coating of nanoparticles with hydrophilic and biocompatible ligands is also possible in one-pot after lowering the reaction temperature to ~100 °C [3]. A general reaction scheme for this is shown in Figure 3.1. Briefly, Ln(III) precursor (generally, halide or nitrate) is added to the TEG. The reaction mixture is magnetically stirred under atmospheric conditions until it is completely dissolved in the TEG at 80 to 100 °C. Then the NaOH solution dissolved in the TEG is added to the precursor solution. The reaction temperature is elevated to 180 to 200 °C. The reaction continues for several hours for nanoparticle formation.

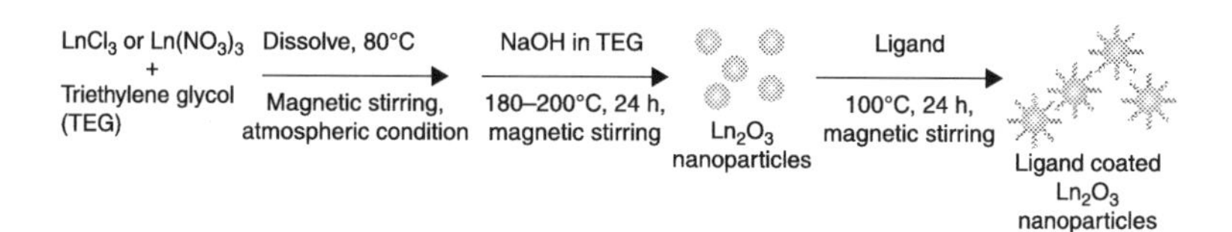

Figure 3.1 The high temperature polyol method

3.1.2 Low temperature polyol method

The above high temperature polyol method can be easily modified into the low temperature polyol method (Figure 3.2), where the reaction can be carried out at ~80 °C instead of 180 to 200 °C. To accomplish this, after adding NaOH solution into the precursor solution at 80 to 100 °C, a H_2O_2 aqueous solution is slowly dripped into the reaction solution using a syringe, while the reaction solution is magnetically stirred for several hours for nanoparticle formation. An advantage of this low temperature polyol method over the high temperature polyol method is that particle diameter can be somewhat reduced compared to those produced by the high temperature polyol method.

3.1.3 Other methods to produce gadolinium oxide (Gd_2O_3) nanoparticles

Gd_2O_3 nanoparticles have been synthesized by various researchers using different methods. Gd_2O_3 nanoparticles with particle diameters of 18 to 66 nm have been synthesized by annealing $Gd(OH)_3$ nanorods from 773 to 1273 K in either air or argon atmosphere [4]. Those with particle diameter of 20 nm have been synthesized by the reverse

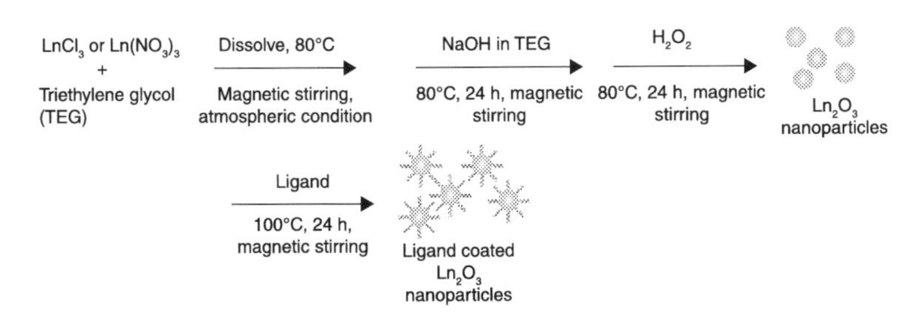

Figure 3.2 The low temperature polyol method

micelle method [5]. In this method, $GdCl_3.6H_2O$ is reacted with NH_4OH in the presence of sodium bis(2-ethylhexyl) sulfosuccinate (AOT) as a surfactant in isooctane/water. Gd_2O_3 nanoparticles with particle diameters of 2.3 nm inside single-wall carbon nanohorns (SWNH) with diameters of 2 to 5 nm, have been synthesized by annealing Gd-acetates encapsulated inside SWNHs at 700 °C in argon flow for 1 hour [6]. Gd(III) clusters with a size of 1 × 2–5 nm have been synthesized inside ultra-short SWNTs (US-SWNT) (20–80 nm long and 3–10 nm thick) that were obtained by cutting SWNTs after fluorination and pyrolysis at 1000 °C under inert atmosphere [7]. In that experiment, the US-SWNTs were loaded with Gd(III) ions by soaking and sonicating them in deionized water (pH = 7) containing $GdCl_3$.

3.2 Surface coating

3.2.1 Possible ligand

Surface coating of synthesized ultrasmall lanthanide oxide nanoparticles is essential for biomedical applications, because they are toxic and insoluble in water. Biocompatibility and water-solubility are necessary for biomedical applications. It is known that free Gd(III) can cause disease such as nephrogenic systemic fibrosis (NSF) [8]. Therefore, ultrasmall lanthanide oxide nanoparticles should be completely coated with hydrophilic and biocompatible ligand.

Ligand coated nanoparticles should be stable in water (i.e. no precipitation, no aggregation, and no decomposition). The stabilizing mechanism of nanoparticles by ligand depends on their molecular weight and surface charge. In general, two stabilizing mechanisms of surface coated nanoparticles in solution are known. One is a surface charge repulsion between ligand coated nanoparticles and the other is a steric hindrance between ligand coated nanoparticles [9]. Large ligands such as polymers are efficient for a steric hindrance, whereas small ligands are not. Therefore, small ligands should have a high surface charge for charge repulsion. As the molecular weight of the ligand increases, water solubility of surface coated nanoparticles generally increases. However, the hydrodynamic diameter also increases accordingly, which might not be ideal for renal excretion.

Various ligands have been used for surface coating. To be coated onto nanoparticles, the ligand should have functional groups such as –COOH, $–NH_2$, -SH, and –OH. The –COOH can be strongly conjugated to a nanoparticle through electrostatic interaction with a surface metal ion [2,10–12]. Examples include PEG diacid, D-glucuronic acid, poly acrylic acid (PAA), and folic acid (Figure 3.3). Ligands with low molecular weights ($M < 1000$ emu) include D-glucuronic acid, lactobionic acid, and polyethylene glycol (PEG) diacid. Polymersincludedextran[13],PAA[14],polyvinylpyrrolidone

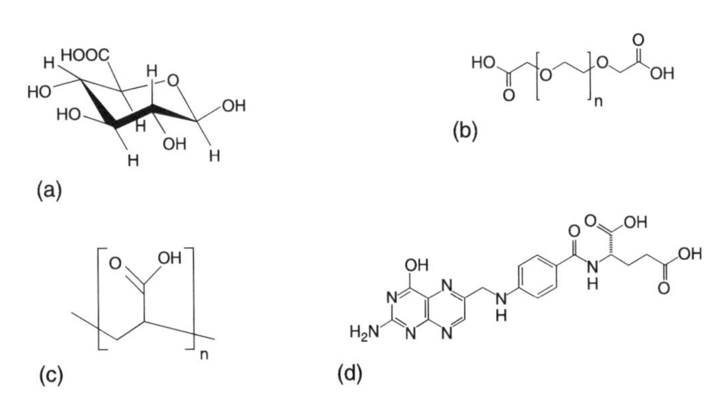

Figure 3.3 Various ligands with –COOH group: (a) D-glucuronic acid; (b) PEG diacid; (c) PAA; and (d) folic acid

(PVP) [15], and polyethyleneimine (PEI) [16]. Biological large molecules, such as bovine serum albumin (BSA) [17] and liposome [18], can be also used for surface coating. Gd_2O_3 nanoparticles can be coated with silica using tetraethylorthosilicate (TEOS) and then further functionalized by PEG diacid [19]. Since the core Gd_2O_3 nanoparticles are completely protected by a silica shell, liberation of free Gd(III) from the core can be minimized.

3.2.2 One-pot ligand coating after nanoparticle formation

Surface coating of nanoparticles with ligand can be done in one-pot. Ligand is added to the reaction solution after synthesis of nanoparticles (Figure 3.1). For surface coating of nanoparticles, the reaction temperature is lowered to ~100 °C and then biocompatible and water-soluble ligand is added to the nanoparticle solution. The reaction mixture is magnetically stirred for more than 6 hours. After surface coating, the solution is cooled to room temperature and then washed with three-times distilled water. The half volume of a sample solution can be used to prepare a sample solution in the three-times distilled water for imaging experiments such as MRI, CT, and FI. The remaining half volume can be subjected to a powder form by drying it in air.

3.2.3 One-pot ligand coating before nanoparticle formation

Another method to synthesize ligand coated ultrasmall lanthanide oxide nanoparticles is as follows. Both ligand and precursor are added to the solvent. In this case, a metal complex is formed and then surface coated nanoparticles are

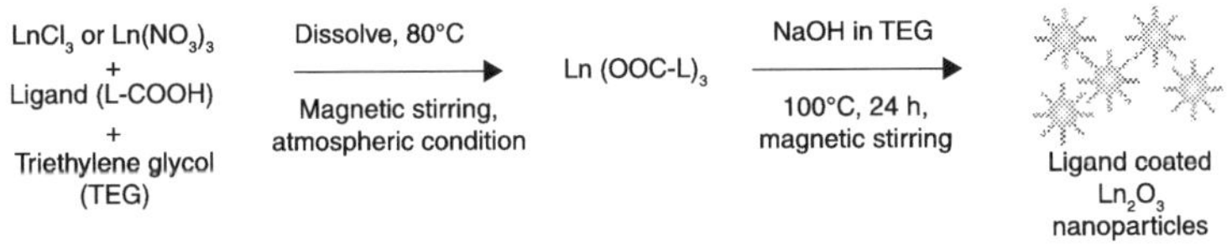

$LnCl_3$ or $Ln(NO_3)_3$ + Ligand (L-COOH) + Triethylene glycol (TEG) —Dissolve, 80°C; Magnetic stirring, atmospheric condition→ Ln $(OOC\text{-}L)_3$ —NaOH in TEG; 100°C, 24 h, magnetic stirring→ Ligand coated Ln_2O_3 nanoparticles

Figure 3.4 Nanoparticle synthesis through a complex formation

produced after adding NaOH to the reaction solution (Figure 3.4). Nanoparticles produced by this method are smaller in diameter than those produced by the high and low temperature polyol methods shown in Figures 3.1 and 3.2, respectively. In addition, surface coating seems to be better in the present case.

3.3 Other lanthanide nano-systems

3.3.1 Lanthanide hydroxide nanorods

As mentioned above, lanthanide hydroxide nanorods are produced instead of lanthanide oxide nanoparticles when Ln(III) reacts with NaOH in water [1]. The crystal structure is hexagonal and the morphology is rod-like. An example of $Gd(OH)_3$ nanorods are shown in Figure 3.5; the suggested reaction mechanism for this is

$$\text{Ln(III) (aq)} + 3\text{OH}^- \text{ (aq)} \rightarrow \text{Ln(OH)}_3 \qquad [3.2]$$

3.3.2 Other gadolinium containing nano-systems

A variety of gadolinium containing nano-systems have been synthesized. These include:

- gadolinium carbonate ($Gd_2O(CO_3)_2.H_2O$) nanoparticle [20];
- $Gd_2O(CO_3)_2.H_2O$/silica/Au hybrid nanoparticle [21];
- $GdPO_4$ nanorod [22];
- GdF_3 nanoparticle [23];
- $NaGdF_4$ nanoparticle [24];
- Eu(III) doped Gd_2O_3 nanoparticle [25];
- Tb(III) doped Gd_2O_3 nanoparticle [26];
- Gd(III) doped CdSe nanoparticle [27];

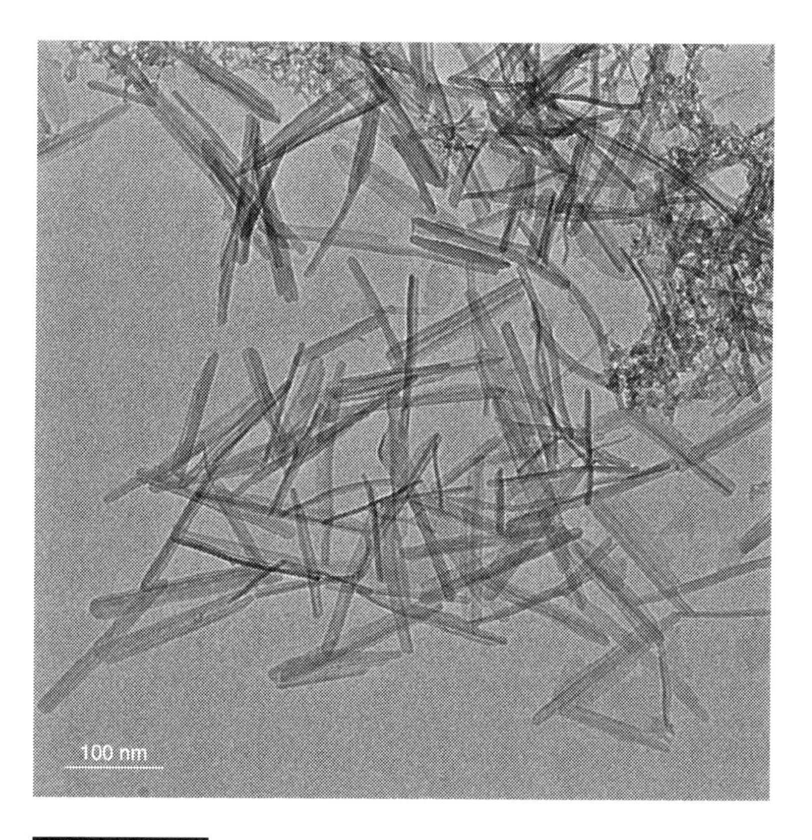

Figure 3.5 A TEM image of $Gd(OH)_3$ nanorods

- $GdPO_4$:Eu(III) hollow sphere [28];
- Yb(III)/Er(III) doped Gd_2O_3 hollow sphere [29]; and
- Gd-nanoscale metal organic framework (NMOF) [30].

These nano-systems have also shown large longitudinal water proton relaxivities and as a result, positive or brighter contrast enhancements in T_1 MR images.

3.4 References

1. Chang, C, and Mao, D. (2007), 'Thermal dehydration kinetics of a rare earth hydroxide, $Gd(OH)_3$', *Int. J. Chem. Kinet.*, 39: 75–81.
2. Söderlind, F., Pedersen, H., Petoral, R.M., Käll, P.-O. and Uvdal, K. (2005), 'Synthesis and characterization of Gd_2O_3 nanocrystals functionalized by organic acids', *J. Colloid Interface Sci.*, 288: 140–8.
3. Park, J.Y., Baek, M.J., Choi, E.S., Woo, S., Kim, J.H. et al. (2009), 'Paramagnetic ultrasmall gadolinium oxide nanoparticles as advanced T_1 MRI contrast agent: account for large longitudinal relaxivity, optimal particle diameter, and *in vivo* T_1 MR images', *ACS Nano*, 3: 3663–9.
4. Sakai, N., Zhu, L., Kurokawa, A., Takeuchi, H., Yano, S. et al. (2012), 'Synthesis of Gd_2O_3 nanoparticles for MRI contrast agents', *J. Phys.: Conf. Ser.*, 352 012008 (6 pages).
5. Roberts, D., Zhu, W.L., Frommen, C.M. and Rosenzweig, Z. (2000), 'Synthesis of gadolinium oxide magnetoliposomes for magnetic resonance imaging', *J. Appl. Phys.*, 87: 6208–10.
6. Miyawaki, J., Yudasaka, M., Imai, H., Yorimitsu, H., Isobe, H. et al. (2006), 'Synthesis of ultrafine Gd_2O_3

nanoparticles inside single-wall carbon nanohorns', *J. Phys. Chem. B*, 110: 5179–81.

7. Sitharaman, B., Kissell, K.R., Hartman, K.B., Tran, L.A., Baikalov, A. et al. (2005), 'Superparamagnetic gadonanotubes are high-performance MRI contrast agents', *Chem. Comm.*, 3915–17.
8. Thomsen, H.S. (2006), 'Nephrogenic systemic fibrosis: a serious late adverse reaction to gadodiamide', *Eur. Radiol.*, 16: 2619–21.
9. Kraynov, A. and Müller, T.E. (2011), 'Concepts for the Stabilization of Metal Nanoparticles in Ionic Liquids', in: Scott Handy (Ed.), *Applications of Ionic Liquids in Science and Technology*, Rijeka, Croatia: InTech.
10. Duckworth, O.W. and Martin, S.T. (2001), 'Surface complexation and dissolution of hematite by C_1-C_6 dicarboxylic acids at pH = 5.0', *Geochim. Cosmochim. Acta*, 65: 4289–301.
11. Hug, S.J. and Bahnemann, D. (2006), 'Infrared spectra of oxalate, malonate and succinate adsorbed on the aqueous surface of rutile, anatase and lepidocrocite measured with *in situ* ATR-FTIR', *J. Electron Spectro. Related Phenomena*, 150: 208–19.
12. Mendive, C.B., Bredow, T., Blesa, M.A. and Bahnemann, D.W. (2006), 'ATR-FTIR measurements and quantum chemical calculations concerning the adsorption and photoreaction of oxalic acid on TiO_2', *Phys. Chem. Chem. Phys.*, 8: 3232–47.
13. McDonald, M.A. and Watkin, K.L. (2006), 'Investigations into the physicochemical properties of dextran small particulate gadolinium oxide nanoparticles', *Acad. Radiol.*, 13: 421–7.
14. Cheung, E.N.M., Alvares, R.D.A., Oakden, W., Chaudhary, R., Hill, M.L. et al. (2010), 'Polymer-

stabilized lanthanide fluoride nanoparticle aggregates as contrast agents for magnetic resonance imaging and computed tomography', *Chem. Mater.*, 22: 4728–39.

15. Johnson, N.J.J., Oakden, W., Stanisz, G.J., Prosser, R.S. and van Veggel, F.C.J.M. (2011) 'Size-tunable, ultrasmall $NaGdF_4$ nanoparticles: insight into their T_1 MRI contrast enhancement', *Chem. Mater.*, 23: 3714–22.
16. Xu, W., Park, J.Y., Kattel, K., Ahmad, M.W., Bony, B.A. et al. (2012), 'Fluorescein-polyethyleneimine coated gadolinium oxide nanoparticles as T_1 magnetic resonance imaging (MRI) – cell labeling (CL) dual agents', *RSC Adv.*, 2: 10907–15.
17. McDonald, M.A. and Watkin, K.L. (2003), 'Small particulate gadolinium oxide and gadolinium albumin microspheres as multimodal contrast and therapeutic agents', *Invest. Radiol.*, 38: 305–10.
18. Roberts, D., Zhu, W.L., Frommen, C.M. and Rosenzweig, Z. (2000), 'Synthesis of gadolinium oxide magnetoliposomes for magnetic resonance imaging', *J. Appl. Phys.*, 87: 6208–10.
19. Bridot, J.-L., Faure, A.-C., Laurent, S., Rivière, C., Billotey, C. et al. (2007), 'Hybrid gadolinium oxide nanoparticles: multimodal contrast agents for *in vivo* imaging', *J. Am. Chem. Soc.*, 129: 5076–84.
20. Li, I.-F., Su, C.-H., Sheu, H.-S., Chiu, H.-C., Lo, Y.-W. et al. (2008), '$Gd_2O(CO_3)_2.H_2O$ particles and the corresponding Gd_2O_3: Synthesis and applications of magnetic resonance contrast agents and template particles for hollow spheres and hybrid composites', *Adv. Funct. Mater.*, 18: 766–76.
21. Hu, K.-W., Jhang, F.-Y., Su, C.-H. and Yeh, C.-S. (2009), 'Fabrication of $Gd_2O(CO_3)_2.H_2O$/silica/gold hybrid particles as a bifunctional agent for MR imaging

and photothermal destruction of cancer cells', *J. Mater. Chem.*, 19: 2147–53.

22. Hifumi, H., Yamaoka, S., Tanimoto, A., Citterio, D. and Suzuki, K. (2006), 'Gadolinium-based hybrid nanoparticles as a positive MR contrast agent', *J. Am. Chem. Soc.*, 128: 15090–1.
23. Evanics, F., Diamente, P.R., van Veggel, F.C.J.M., Stanisz, G.J. and Prosser, R.S. (2006), 'Water-soluble GdF_3 and GdF_3/LaF_3 nanoparticles-physical characterization and NMR relaxation properties', *Chem. Mater.*, 18: 2499–505.
24. Johnson, N.J.J., Oakden, W., Stanisz, G.J., Prosser, R.S. and van Veggel, F.C.J.M. (2011), 'Size-tunable, ultrasmall $NaGdF_4$ nanoparticles: insight into their T_1 MRI contrast enhancement', *Chem. Mater.*, 23: 3714–22.
25. Shi, Z., Neoh, K.G., Kang, E.T., Shuter, B. and Wang, S.-C. (2010), 'Bifunctional Eu^{3+}-doped Gd_2O_3 nanoparticles as a luminescent and T_1 contrast agent for stem cell labeling', *Contrast Media Mol. Imaging*, 5: 1–7.
26. Petoral, R.M., Söderlind, F., Klasson, A., Suska, A., Fortin, M.A. et al. (2009), 'Synthesis and characterization of Tb^{3+}-doped Gd_2O_3 nanocrystals: a bifunctional material with combined fluorescent labeling and MRI contrast agent properties', *J. Phys. Chem. C*, 113: 6913–20.
27. Li, I.-F. and Yeh, C.-S. (2010), 'Synthesis of Gd doped CdSe nanoparticles for potential optical and MR imaging applications', *J. Mater. Chem.*, 20: 2079–81.
28. Zhang, L., Yin, M., You, H., Yang, M., Song, Y. and Huang, Y. (2011), 'Multifunctional $GdPO_4$:Eu^{3+} hollow spheres: synthesis and magnetic and luminescent properties', *Inorg. Chem.*, 50: 10608–13.

29. Tian, G., Gu, Z., Liu, X., Zhou, L., Yin, W. et al. (2011), 'Facile fabrication of rare-earth-doped Gd_2O_3 hollow spheres with up-conversion luminescence, magnetic resonance, and drug delivery properties', *J. Phys. Chem. C*, 115: 23790–6.
30. Rocca, J.D. and Lin, W. (2010), 'Nanoscale metal-organic frameworks: magnetic resonance imaging contrast agents and beyond', *Eur. J. Inorg. Chem.*, 24: 3725–34.

Characterization

DOI: 10.1533/9780081000694.43

Abstract: This chapter discusses characterization of physical, chemical, and imaging properties of ligand coated ultrasmall lanthanide oxide nanoparticles using various techniques. These include measurement of particle diameter, hydrodynamic diameter, crystal structure, surface coating, cytotoxicity, magnetic properties, water proton relaxivities, map images, biodistribution, and fluorescent properties.

Key words: characterization, physical property, chemical property, imaging property.

4.1 Introduction

The synthesized surface coated ultrasmall lanthanide oxide nanoparticles should be characterized by using various techniques. These include:

- measurements of particle diameter and morphology using a high resolution transmission electron microscope (HRTEM);
- crystal structure using an X-ray diffraction (XRD) spectrometer;

- ligand surface coating using a Fourier transform infrared (FT-IR) absorption spectrometer;
- ligand surface coating amount using a thermogravimetric analyzer (TGA);
- magnetic properties using a superconducting quantum interference device (SQUID) magnetometer;
- hydrodynamic diameter using a dynamic light scattering (DLS) particle size analyzer;
- lanthanide metal ion concentration in an aqueous sample solution using an inductively coupled plasma atomic emission spectrometer (ICPAES);
- *in vitro* cytotoxicity using an assay kit and luminometer;
- biodistribution using an ICPAES and a HRTEM;
- fluorescent properties using a photoluminescence (PL) spectrometer; and
- relaxivity and map images using a magnetic resonance imaging (MRI) scanner.

4.2 Particle diameter and morphology

The particle diameter and morphology are very important for MRI contrast agents. Since a MRI contrast agent is administered into the body through intravenous injection, particle diameter should be as small as possible for renal excretion. Lanthanide ions (i.e. Ln(III)) are toxic and thus cannot be digested inside the body, unlike iron oxide nanoparticles that can be digested into various forms such as ferritin and hemoglobin, because iron is an essential element in the body. For renal excretion, spherical morphology is preferred to other morphologies such as rod and square, because a spherical nanoparticle can be more easily passed through a capillary vessel, whereas other morphologies could become stuck inside a capillary vessel.

Both particle diameter and morphology can be measured using a HRTEM (Figure 4.1). A HRTEM with acceleration voltages of 200 keV is enough to measure particle diameter

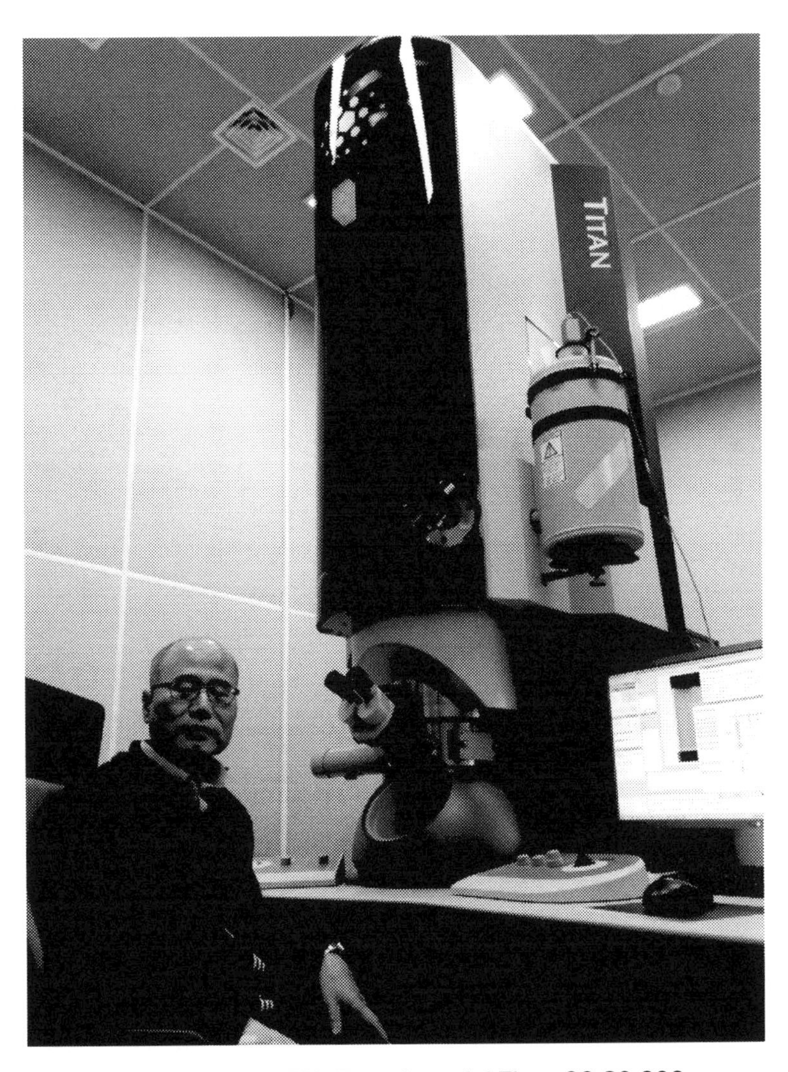

Figure 4.1 A HRTEM (Tecnai, model Titan G2 80 200 ChemiSTEM) and the author (GHL)

as small as 1.0 nm with lattice resolution. One example of a HRTEM image of ultrasmall gadolinium oxide nanoparticles is shown in Figure 4.2. The figure shows that the nanoparticles are aggregated and the particle diameter ranges from 1 to 3 nm. A single nanoparticle is indicated with a dotted circle. However, a HRTEM with an acceleration voltage of 300 keV, or a high voltage electron microscope (HVEM) with an acceleration voltage of 1.2 MeV, can be used to measure particle diameters of less than 1.0 nm.

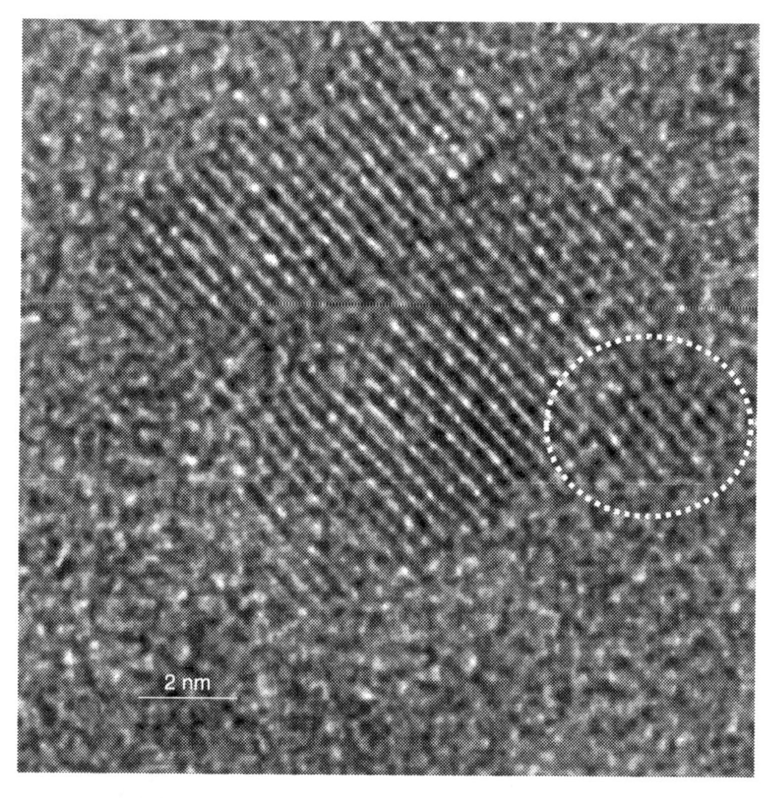

Figure 4.2 A HRTEM image of D-glucuronic acid coated ultrasmall gadolinium oxide nanoparticles. A single nanoparticle is indicated with a dotted circle

In order to measure the particle diameter, hydrophilic ligand coated nanoparticles dispersed in water or ethanol are dropped onto a copper grid using a micro-dispenser. The solvent used should be evaporated from the sample in air before loading it inside the HRTEM.

A HRTEM equipped with an energy-dispersive X-ray spectrometer (the so-called EDX or EDS) can be used for elemental analysis. Furthermore, an elemental mapping of two-dimensional (2-D) distribution of elements can be measured using an EDX or electron energy loss spectroscopy (EELS) in scanning mode (i.e. STEM). This technique is known as high-angle annular dark-field imaging (HAADF). From elemental mapping the core-shell structure, hetero-structure, surface oxidation, and ligand coating of nanoparticle can be investigated. For elemental mapping of individual nanoparticles, particle diameter should be practically larger than 5 nm to obtain a sufficient signal to noise ratio. Otherwise, signals are too low to observe an elemental map image of each nanoparticle.

4.3 Crystal structure

The crystal structure of nanoparticles can be measured using an XRD spectrometer. The crystal structure is a finger-print of identifying nanoparticle species. The XRD pattern of a nanoparticle is taken using a powder sample. The particle diameter (d) can be roughly estimated by measuring the full width at half maximum (FWHM) of the peaks and using the Scherrer's formula [1]:

$$d = \frac{K\lambda}{\beta \cos\theta} \quad [4.1]$$

in which K is the shape factor (= 0.89), λ is the X-ray wavelength, β is the FWHM, and θ is the Bragg angle that is estimated from the peak position (= 2θ)). Here, the FWHM and 2θ are obtained from Lorentzian function fitting to an observed peak. As d decreases, the FWHM becomes broader. If d is less than 2 nm, the nanoparticle could be poorly crystallized. Quasi-crystal structures such as decahedrons, octahedrons, and icosahedrons, could appear [2]. For example, Au_{55} has an icosahedron structure [3]. If d is less than 1 nm, an amorphous pattern could appear. One example of an XRD pattern of D-glucuronic acid coated ultrasmall gadolinium oxide nanoparticles is shown in Figure 4.3. The figure shows that the XRD pattern is very broad and looks amorphous. However, sharp peaks corresponding to a cubic structure of Gd_2O_3 appear, as shown in Figure 4.3, after annealing of up to 700 °C due to crystal growth.

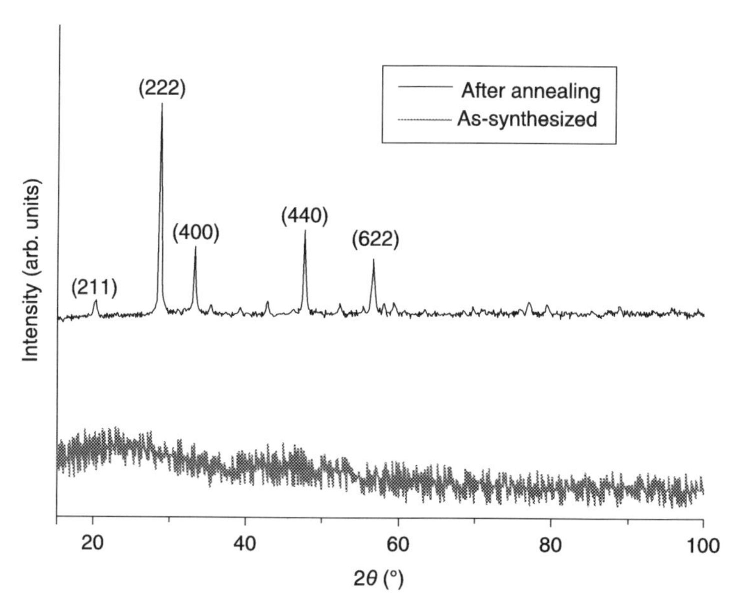

Figure 4.3 XRD patterns of D-glucuronic acid coated ultrasmall gadolinium oxide nanoparticles: as-synthesized (bottom) and after annealing up to 700 °C (top)

Pure metals and metal oxides typically have crystal structures such as body-centered cubic (bcc), face-centered cubic (fcc), and hexagonal close packed (hcp). Tetragonal, monoclinic, and triclinic crystal structures are occasionally observed. These crystal structures are identified by taking an XRD pattern. The cell constants (or lattice constants or lattice parameters) (a, b, c, α, β, γ) are then determined using the following formula in the case of cubic (Equation 4.2), tetragonal (Equation 4.3), and hcp (Equation 4.4) [1]:

$$\text{Cubic structure: } \frac{\sin^2\theta}{(h^2+k^2+l^2)} = \frac{\lambda^2}{4a^2}, \quad [4.2]$$

$$\text{Tetragonal structure: } \frac{4\sin^2\theta}{\lambda^2} = \frac{h^2+k^2}{a^2} + \frac{l^2}{c^2}, \quad [4.3]$$

$$\text{Hexagonal structure: } \frac{4\sin^2\theta}{\lambda^2} = \frac{4}{3} \times \frac{h^2+k^2+hk}{a^2} + \frac{l^2}{c^2} \quad [4.4]$$

Different formulas should be used for other structures [1].

Three forms of lanthanide oxides exist. These are hexagonal $Ln(OH)_3$, monoclinic LnOOH, and cubic Ln_2O_3 [4], and the corresponding morphologies are rod, rod, and spherical. As mentioned above, $Ln(OH)_3$ is exclusively formed when Ln(III) reacts with NaOH in water, because of a high dehydration energy from $Ln(OH)_3$ to Ln_2O_3 [4]. However, $Ln(OH)_3$ transforms into LnOOH and then into Ln_2O_3 by calcination. Therefore, Ln^{3+} should react with NaOH in polyol solvent at elevated temperatures to obtain Ln_2O_3 nanoparticles, as already mentioned in Chapter 3 [5].

4.4 Hydrodynamic diameter (a)

The hydrodynamic diameter of surface coated nanoparticles is measured using a DLS particle size analyzer. For biomedical applications, the hydrodynamic diameter is more important than particle diameter measured from a HRTEM. The hydrodynamic diameter is generally larger than particle diameter because of the presence of ligand and solvated water molecules. It is known that nanoparticles with hydrodynamic diameters of less than 5 nm can be excreted from the body through the renal system [6]. Since most nanoparticles are toxic, complete renal excretion is a pre-requisite to clinical applications.

Hydrodynamic diameter distribution follows a log-normal distribution similar to particle diameter distribution. Therefore, an average hydrodynamic diameter can be obtained by fitting the observed hydrodynamic diameters to a log-normal function. In the case of monodispersed nanoparticles, the hydrodynamic diameter distribution will be very narrow. These hydrodynamic diameters depend on ligands; for large ligands such as polymers, the hydrodynamic diameters are large, whereas for small ligands the hydrodynamic diameters are small. However, the colloidal stability increases with increasing ligand size, because the steric hindrance increases accordingly. This implies that ligand with proper size should be used for the surface coating to reduce a hydrodynamic diameter for renal excretion. Nanoparticles coated with ligand with a strong surface charge can strongly repel each other. Therefore, surface coating with ligand with a small size but a high surface charge will be extremely useful for biomedical applications. One example of a DLS pattern of D-glucuronic acid coated gadolinium oxide nanoparticles is shown in Figure 4.4. The figure shows that the hydrodynamic diameter distribution is narrow and the average hydrodynamic diameter is 7.3 nm.

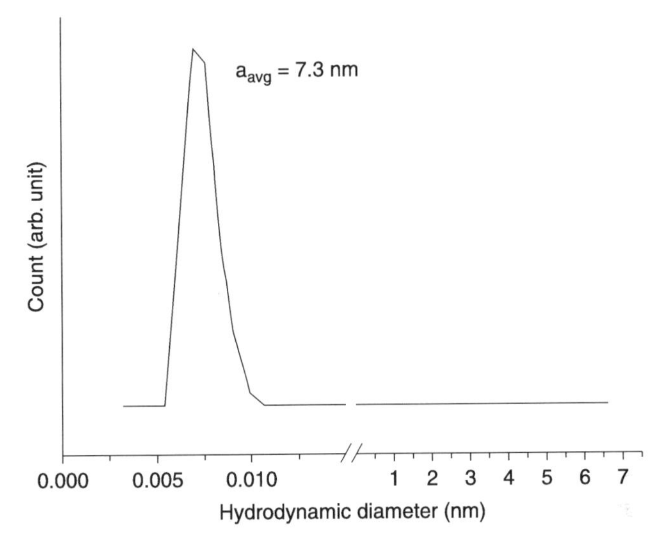

Figure 4.4 A DLS pattern of D-glucuronic acid coated ultrasmall gadolinium oxide nanoparticles

4.5 Surface coating confirmation

Surface coating can be analyzed by recording a FT-IR absorption spectrum of surface coated nanoparticle. In order to record a FT-IR absorption spectrum, a powder sample is mixed with KBr and then a pallet is prepared. The spectrum is scanned between 400 and 4000 cm^{-1}. In order to confirm the surface coating, a FT-IR absorption spectrum should be compared with that of a free ligand. From the comparison, the surface coating can be confirmed from characteristic vibrational peaks of the ligand. The absorption peaks from the ligand, such as C–H stretch at ~2900 cm^{-1} and C=O stretch at ~1600 cm^{-1}, will be observed in the case of the ligand with -COOH. Here, the C=O stretch of the surface coated ligand is generally red-shifted by ~100 cm^{-1} from ~1700 cm^{-1} of a free –COOH, because the –COOH group is chemically conjugated to a nanoparticle.

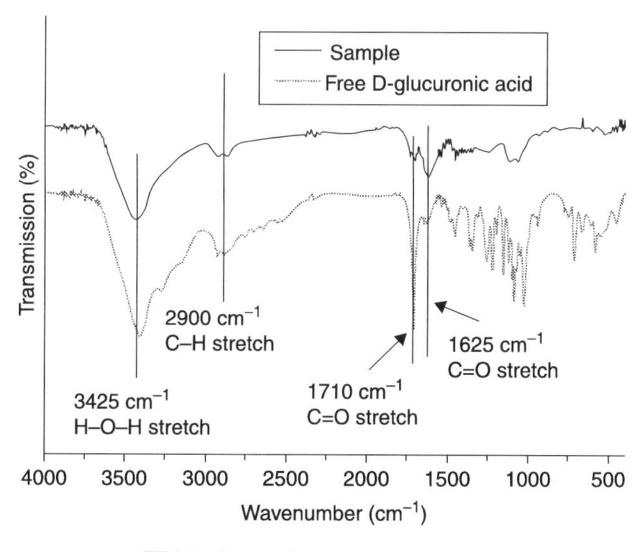

Figure 4.5 FT-IR absorption spectra of D-glucuronic acid coated gadolinium oxide nanoparticle and a free D-glucuronic acid

Figure 4.5 shows an example of FT-IR absorption spectra of D-glucuronic acid coated gadolinium oxide nanoparticle and a free D-glucuronic acid. The figure shows that the C-H stretch at 2900 cm^{-1} and the C=O stretch at 1625 cm^{-1} are observed due to surface coated D-glucuronic acid. Here, the C=O stretch is red-shifted by 85 cm^{-1} from that of a free D-glucuronic acid, confirming that the –COOH group of D-glucuronic acid is chemically conjugated to a Gd_2O_3 nanoparticle. Similar red shifts had been observed in gadolinium oxide nanoparticles coated with various ligands with the –COOH group [5].

4.6 Surface coating amount

The nanoparticles should be sufficiently coated with ligand for biocompatibility and water-solubility. The coating amount of ligand can be measured by recording a TGA curve in air flow. Most organic ligands burn out below 400 °C and thus a temperature scan up to 700 °C will be enough. A powder sample is loaded to TGA and a TGA curve is scanned between room temperature and 700 °C. A slight mass drop between room temperature and 100 to 115 °C is due to moisture desorption. Above this, a mass drop is due to ligand burning. After all the ligand has burned, a flat TGA curve is obtained, because of the remaining metal oxide nanoparticles.

Figure 4.6 shows a TGA curve of D-glucuronic acid coated gadolinium oxide nanoparticles. As shown in the figure, an initial drop of 15% corresponds to water desorption between room temperature and 105 °C, the next drop of 38% between 105 and 450 °C corresponds to burning of D-glucuronic acid, and the remaining 47% above 450 °C corresponds to the Gd_2O_3 nanoparticle. After TGA, the remaining sample is a pure metal oxide nanoparticle with increased particle

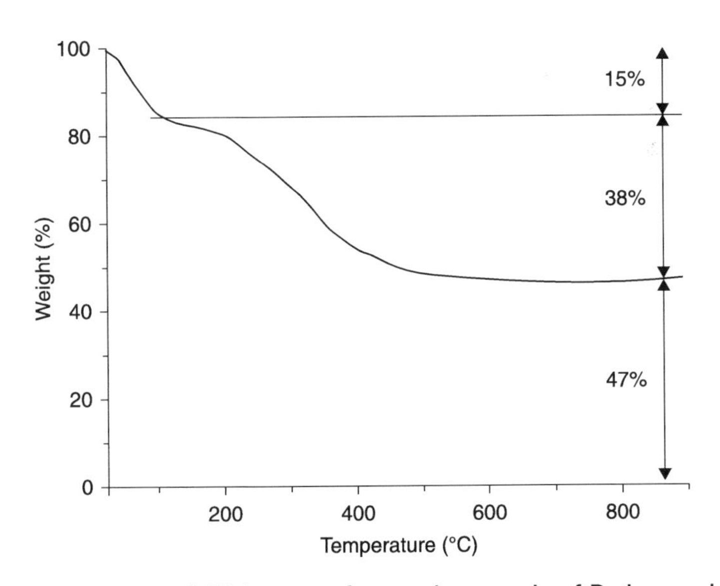

Figure 4.6 A TGA curve of a powder sample of D-glucuronic acid coated gadolinium oxide nanoparticles

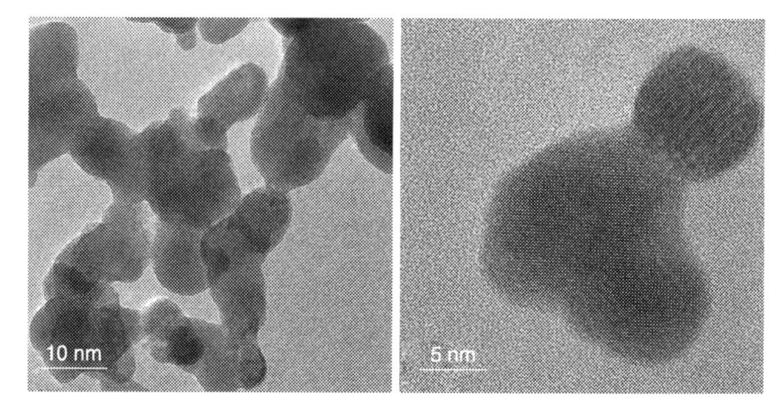

Figure 4.7 TEM images of D-glucuronic acid coated gadolinium oxide nanoparticles after TGA at 5 and 10 nm scales, showing the particle growth compared to as-prepared nanoparticles shown in Figure 4.2

diameter [7]. This can be confirmed by TEM images (Figure 4.7), which show the particle diameter to have grown during annealing. This particle size growth can be confirmed by examining the particle diameter of the as-prepared nanoparticles (Figure 4.2) and comparing it with that after TGA (Figure 4.7). For sufficient surface coating, the ligand coating amount should be more than 20% in weight percent. The surface coating amount in weight percent can be converted into grafting density, corresponding to the number of ligand molecules grafted onto a unit surface area of a nanoparticle. This number should be larger than $1.0/nm^2$ for there to be enough surface coating [8].

4.7 Magnetic properties

Magnetic properties of a MRI contrast agent are very important. They should possess large magnetic moments, because water proton relaxivities depend on the magnetic moment. Nanoparticles made of metal ions with large and pure electron spin magnetic moments can strongly accelerate the longitudinal water proton (i.e. T_1) relaxation, whereas nanoparticles with a large total magnetic moment can strongly accelerate the transverse water proton (i.e. T_2) relaxation.

Magnetic properties of nanoparticles can be characterized by recording magnetization (M) versus applied field (H) (i.e. a M-H curve) and zero-field-cooled (ZFC) and field-cooled (FC) M versus temperature (T) (i.e. ZFC/FC M-T curves). The ZFC/FC M-T curves are generally recorded at an applied field of 100 oersted (Oe) for T between 5 and 300 K, while a M-H curve is scanned for H between −5 and 5 tesla and at T = 5 and 300 K. These curves are recorded using a SQUID magnetometer.

From both M-H and M-T curves, magnetism (superparamagnetism, paramagnetism, ferromagnetism, antiferromagnetism, and nonmagnetism), saturation magnetization (M_s), coercivity (H_c), remanence (M_r), and phase transition temperature such as Curie (T_C), Niel (T_N), and blocking (T_B) temperatures can be determined. Ultrasmall lanthanide oxide nanoparticles show paramagnetism, like bulk materials [7]. Therefore, they do not show saturation magnetization but decent magnetization at room temperature, because of a large magnetic moment of lanthanide ion. However, at a low temperature, they show a very large and nearly saturated magnetization, which is larger than those (>50 emu/g) of superparamagnetic iron oxide (SPIO) nanoparticles [7].

Molecules cannot have a large magnetization at room temperature. Therefore, only nanoparticles can be used as T_2 MRI contrast agents. Ultrasmall lanthanide metal oxide nanoparticles (Ln = Dy, Ho, Tb, Er, etc.) have decent magnetizations at room temperature and thus, appreciable r_2 values have been observed [7]. Since the r_2 value is proportional to the square of the applied MR field, their r_2 value will be very large or even larger than that of SPIO nanoparticle at high MR fields such as 7 tesla. Therefore, they are potential T_2 MRI contrast agents at high MR fields.

Ultrasmall gadolinium oxide nanoparticles have been intensively studied as potential T_1 MRI contrast agents, because Gd^{3+} is the ion with highest spin magnetic moment ($s = 7/2$) in the periodic table arising from 7 unpaired 4f-electrons of Gd^{3+}. Ultrasmall gadolinium oxide nanoparticles have shown a large r_1 value [9]. After intravenous administration, they have shown a clear positive (i.e. brighter) contrast enhancement. Therefore, the ultrasmall gadolinium oxide nanoparticle is a potential T_1 MRI contrast agent.

As an example, a mass corrected ZFC M-T curve at $H = 100$ Oe and M-H curves at $T = 5$ and 300 K are shown in Figure 4.8. These curves are recorded using a powder sample of D-glucuronic acid coated ultrasmall gadolinium oxide nanoparticles. Here, magnetization corresponds to net magnetization of ultrasmall gadolinium oxide nanoparticles in D-glucuronic acid coated ultrasmall gadolinium oxide nanoparticles, because measured magnetization is mass corrected with net mass of ultrasmall gadolinium oxide nanoparticles in D-glucuronic acid coated ultrasmall gadolinium oxide nanoparticles estimated from a TGA curve. The M-H curves at both $T = 5$ and 300 K show that both coercivity and remanance are zero (i.e. no hysteresis). This lack of hysteresis, as well as no magnetic transition down to $T = 3$ K in an ZFC M-T curve, indicates that nanoparticles are paramagnetic down to $T = 3$ K. Paramagnetism had been observed for all lanthanide oxide nanoparticles [7], which is consistent with various reports on bulks [10–16]. Ultrasmall

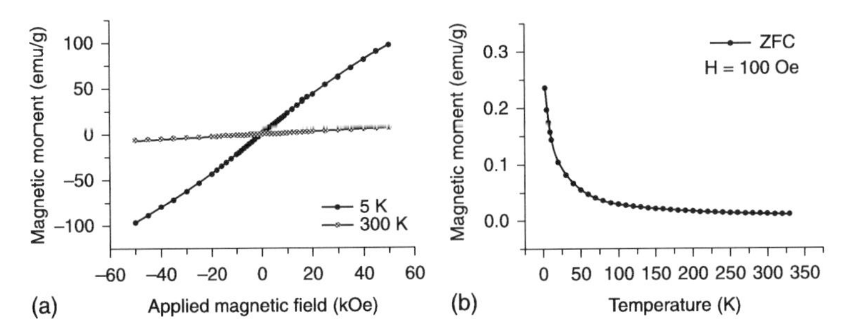

Figure 4.8 Mass corrected M-H curves at T = 5 and 300 K (a) and ZFC M-T curve at H = 100 Oe (b) of a powder sample of D-glucuronic acid coated ultrasmall gadolinium oxide nanoparticles

lanthanide oxide nanoparticles, except for ultrasmall europium oxide nanoparticles, have shown appreciable magnetic moments at room temperature [7]. Their magnetic moments do not drop very far with decreasing particle diameter and by surface coating with ligand. Therefore, ultrasmall lanthanide oxide nanoparticles are promising nanoparticles for use as MRI contrast agents [17].

4.8 Cytotoxicity

The cytotoxicity measurement is necessary before *in vivo* experiments because surface coated nanoparticles should be biocompatible (i.e. non-toxic). In cytotoxicity measurement, the cell viability is generally measured up to 1 mM Ln (Ln = Gd, Dy, Ho, etc.) in an aqueous sample solution. Many cytotoxicity measurement methods have been developed to date. The commonly used methods include:

- adenosine-triphosphate (ATP) test;
- 3-(4,5-*di*methylthiazol-2-yl)-2,5-diphenyltetrazolium bromide (MTT) test;

- lactate dehydrogenase (LDH) test; and
- neutral red method [18–20].

In the ATP test [18], the ATP is essential for live cells and its concentration should be maintained enough for cell viability. However, its concentration rapidly drops when the cell undergoes apoptosis or necrosis. The cell viability after being treated with nanoparticles can be estimated by comparing the ATP concentration of control cells (i.e. the cells not treated with nanoparticles) to that of sample cells treated with nanoparticles. In order to measure ATP concentration, luciferase and D-luciferin are added to the cells. The following reaction occurs with accompanying light emission:

$$\begin{aligned} &\text{ATP} + \text{D-luciferin} + O_2 \xrightarrow{\text{luciferase } Mg^{2+}} \text{oxyluciferin} \\ &+\text{AMP} + PP_1 + CO_2 + \text{light} \end{aligned} \qquad [4.5]$$

The emitted light intensity is proportional to ATP concentration and measured using a luminometer. A CellTiter-Glo Luminescent Cell Viability Assay (Promega, WI, USA) can be used to measure the cellular toxicity of an aqueous sample solution of nanoparticles [7]. One example is shown in Figure 4.9 for an aqueous solution of D-glucuronic acid coated ultrasmall gadolinium oxide nanoparticles using both NCTC1469 (normal mouse hepatocyte cell) and DU145 (human prostate cancer cell) cells. As shown in the figure, D-glucuronic acid coated ultrasmall gadolinium oxide nanoparticles are not toxic up to 200 μM Gd. In general, if *in vitro* cell viability is more than 90% up to 1 mM, the sample is considered to be biocompatible.

In the MTT method [18], the mitochondria that plays a central role in a live cell is indirectly measured. An MTT that is a yellow colored dye is added to the cells. It enters into the mitochondria in a cell, where it is reduced to an insoluble

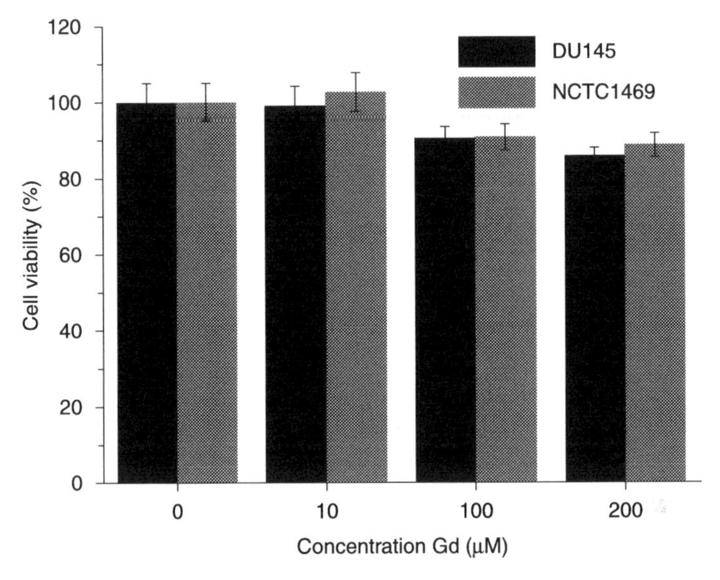

Figure 4.9 Cytotoxicity results of an aqueous sample solution of D-glucuronic acid coated ultrasmall gadolinium oxide nanoparticles using NCTC1469 and DU145 cells

and dark purple formazan by reaction with mitochondrial succinate dehydrogenase. This reduction reaction only occurs in live cells, and so corresponds to a measure of cell viability. The cells are treated with isopropanol organic solvent to extract formazan, which is measured spectrophotometrically at 490 nm.

In the LDH method [19], the LDH that is a soluble cytosolic enzyme is released into the cell culture medium when the cells are dead due to damage of their plasma membranes. Therefore, the concentration of LDH is proportional to the concentration of dead cells. The LDH concentration is indirectly measured. A test solution containing L-lactate, nicotinamide adenine dinucleotide (NAD^+), diaphrose, and 2-(4-iodophenyl)-3-(4-nitrophenyl)-5-phenyl-2H-tetrazolium chloride (tetrazolium salt INT) is added to the cells. The NAD^+ is reduced into NADH in the presence of L-lactate by catalysis of LDH. The tetrazolium salt INT is then reduced into a red formazan product by NADH that is spectrophotometrically measured at 490 nm.

In the neutral red method [20], the neutral red is taken up by live cells only. Therefore, the concentration of dye incorporated into the lysosomes of the cells is proportional to the live cells. The cells are washed several times to remove dye in the culture medium and then treated with an acidified ethanol solution to extract the incorporated dye from the cells. The dye concentration is then measured spectrophotometrically.

4.9 Water proton relaxivity and map image

Longitudinal (r_1) and transverse (r_2) water proton relaxivities (unit: $s^{-1}mM^{-1}$) are physical constants that are used to judge the strength of a sample solution as a MRI contrast agent. These constants can be measured using a MRI scanner. The r_1 and r_2 values should be as large as possible for T_1 and T_2 MRI contrast agents, respectively. The r_2/r_1 ratio is theoretically always greater than one, because the T_1 relaxation always accompanies the T_2 relaxation. Therefore, the r_2/r_1 ratio should be as close as possible to 1.0 for a T_1 MRI contrast agent, whereas it should be as large as possible for a T_2 MRI contrast agent.

In order to estimate r_1 and r_2 values, the longitudinal (T_1) and transverse (T_2) water proton relaxation times (unit: s) are measured as a function of lanthanide (Ln) concentration in an aqueous sample solution. The Ln concentration of a sample solution is determined using an ICPAES, as mentioned before. The measured inverse relaxation times ($1/T_1$ and $1/T_2$) (also known as relaxations (R_1 and R_2)) are then plotted as a function of Ln concentration and then r_1 and r_2 values are obtained from the slopes, respectively. One example using an aqueous sample solution of D-glucuronic acid ultrasmall gadolinium oxide nanoparticle is shown in Figure 4.10. The figure shows, r_1 and r_2 values to be 13.2 and 15.8 $s^{-1}mM^{-1}$, respectively.

Map images are contrast changes as a function of Ln concentration of a sample solution. R_1 and R_2 map images are measured as a function of Ln concentration. Clear dose-dependent contrast changes reflect large relaxivities. That is, a clear dose-dependent contrast change in R_1 map images will be observed if the r_1 value is large. Likewise, a clear dose-dependent contrast change in R_2 map images will be observed if the r_2 value is large. One example is shown in

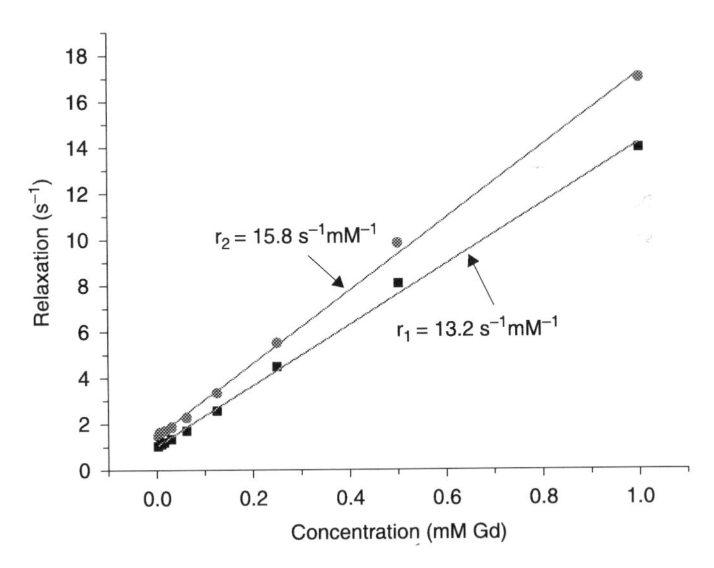

Figure 4.10 Plots of R_1 and R_2 relaxations as a function of Ln concentration for an aqueous solution of D-glucuronic acid ultrasmall gadolinium oxide nanoparticles. The slopes correspond to r_1 and r_2 values, respectively

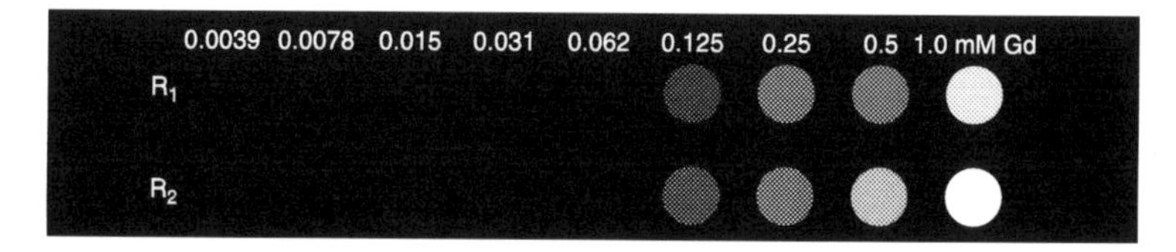

Figure 4.11 R_1 and R_2 map images as a function of Ln concentration for an aqueous solution of D-glucuronic acid coated ultrasmall gadolinium oxide nanoparticle (the same sample in Figure 4.10)

Figure 4.11, using an aqueous solution of D-glucuronic acid coated ultrasmall gadolinium oxide nanoparticles, showing clear dose-dependent contrast enhancements in both R_1 and R_2 map images, as expected from the large r_1 and r_2 values given in Figure 4.10.

4.10 Biodistribution

The biodistribution (i.e. the distribution of nanoparticles in various organs and tissues in the body) of nanoparticles can be determined using an ICPAES. An *in vivo* biodistribution study can be performed by injecting an aqueous sample solution of surface coated ultrasmall lanthanide oxide nanoparticles as a bolus (0.1 mmol/kg) into a mouse tail vein [21]. For consistency, 10 to 20 mice can be used. The mice are anesthetized and euthanized by exsanguination from the vena cava at various time intervals (e.g. 15 min, 3, 6, 12, and 48 h) after intravenous injection. Three to five mice can be used for each time point, in order to obtain average lanthanide (Ln) metal concentrations in various organs and tissues such as blood, liver, heart, kidneys, bladder, and spleen. Ln concentrations are determined by digesting organs and tissues with HNO_3 and H_2O_2 (1:1) at 180 °C for 120 minutes and measuring Ln concentrations in diluted solutions using an ICPAES. The typical detection limit of this method is 0.01 ppm, corresponding to the detection limit of the ICPAES.

4.11 *In vivo* TEM analysis of nanoparticles

For *in vivo* TEM analysis of nanoparticles accumulated in cells of organs and tissues, organs or tissues are removed from a mouse after anesthetizing and euthanizing by exsanguination from the vena cava [22]. The organs are sliced and fixed with polymer. The ultra-thin sections of organ cells in polymer matrix are obtained using an ultramicrotome and then doubly stained with both uranyl acetate and lead citrate solution. Sections are imaged with a TEM at acceleration voltages of 80 to 100 kV. A TEM operated at these voltages is called a bio-TEM.

4.12 Fluorescent properties

Some of the lanthanide elements emit photons in the visible or far infrared region after UV excitation (Chapter 2). Therefore, ultrasmall lanthanide oxide nanoparticles can be used as fluorescent imaging (FI) agents. Especially, ultrasmall lanthanide oxide nanoparticles made of Eu and Tb strongly emit photons in the 600 (red) and 540 (green) nm regions after excitation with UV [23,24]. Furthermore, their fluorescent intensity increases with decreasing particle diameter due to reduced excitation migration to quenching sites that are proportional to particle diameter [25,26]. This property is beneficial to biomedical applications, because

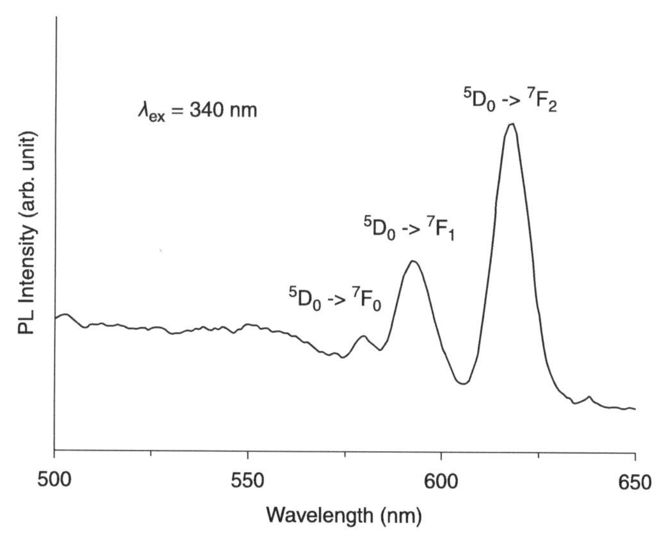

Figure 4.12 A PL spectrum of D-glucuronic acid coated ultrasmall Eu_2O_3 nanoparticles in ethanol using UV excitation wavelength (λ_{ex}) of 340 nm

only ultrasmall nanoparticles can be excreted through the renal system [6].

Fluorescent properties can be measured by recording PL spectra. Nanoparticle solutions are prepared in ethanol at concentrations between 0.1 to 1.0 mM. They are filled into 1.0 mL quartz cell with four clear sides. One example of a PL spectrum of D-glucuronic acid coated ultrasmall Eu_2O_3 nanoparticles is shown in Figure 4.12. The figure shows emission peaks resulting from $^5D_0$ to $^7F_{0,1,2}$ transition in Eu(III). The $^5D_0$ to $^7F_2$ is the most intense transition among them.

4.13 References

1. Cullity, B.D. (1980), *Elements of X-ray Diffraction*, 2nd edn, Reading, UK: Addison-Wesley Publishing Company, Inc.

2. Vogel, W. (1998), 'X-ray diffraction from clusters', *Cryst. Res. Technol.*, 33: 1141–54.
3. Vogel, W., Rosner, B. and Tesche, B. (1993), 'Structural investigations of Au_{55} organometallic complexes by X-ray powder diffraction and transmission electron microscopy', *J. Phys. Chem.*, 97: 11611–16.
4. Chang, C. and Mao, D. (2007), 'Thermal dehydration kinetics of a rare earth hydroxide, $Gd(OH)_3$', *Int. J. Chem. Kinet.*, 39: 75–81.
5. Söderlind, F., Pedersen, H., Petoral, R.M., Käll, P.-O. and Uvdal, K. (2005), 'Synthesis and characterization of Gd_2O_3 nanocrystals functionalized by organic acids', *J. Colloid Interface Sci.*, 288: 140–8.
6. Choi, H.S., Liu, W., Misra, P., Tanaka, E., Zimmer, J.P. et al. (2007), 'Renal clearance of quantum dots', *Nat. Biotechnology*, 25: 1165–70.
7. Kattel, K., Park, J.Y., Xu, W., Kim, H.G., Lee, E.J. et al. (2011), 'A facile synthesis, *in vitro* and *in vivo* MR studies of D-glucuronic acid-coated ultrasmall Ln_2O_3 (Ln = Eu, Gd, Dy, Ho, and Er) nanoparticles as a new potential MRI contrast agent', *ACS Appl. Mater. Interfaces*, 3: 3325–34.
8. Corbierre, M.K., Cameron, N.S. and Lennox, R.B. (2004), 'Polymer-stabilized gold nanoparticles with high grafting densities', *Langmuir*, 20: 2867–73.
9. Park, J.Y., Baek, M.J., Choi, E.S., Woo, S., Kim, J.H. et al. (2009), 'Paramagnetic ultrasmall gadolinium oxide nanoparticles as advanced T_1 MRI contrast agent: account for large longitudinal relaxivity, optimal particle diameter, and *in vivo* T_1 MR images', *ACS Nano*, 3: 3663–9.
10. Arajs, S. and Colvin, R.V. (1964), 'Paramagnetic susceptibility of Eu_2O_3 from 300 to 1300 °K', *J. Appl. Phys.*, 35: 1181–3.

11. Arajs, S. and Colvin, R.V. (1962), 'Magnetic susceptibility of gadolinium and dysprosium sesquioxides at elevated temperatures', *J. Appl. Phys.*, 33: 2517–19.
12. Koehler, W.C., Wollan, E.O. and Wilkinson, M.K. (1958), 'Paramagnetic and nuclear scattering cross-sections of holmium sesquioxide', *Phys. Rev.*, 110: 37–40.
13. Lal, H.B., Pratap, V. and Kumar, A. (1978), 'Magnetic susceptibility of heavy rare-earth sesquioxides', *Pramana*, 10: 409–12.
14. Moon, R.M., Koehler, W.C., Child, H.R and Raubenheimer, L.J. (1968), 'Magnetic structures of Er_2O_3 and Yb_2O_3', *Phys. Rev.*, 176: 722–31.
15. Moon, R.M. and Koehler, W.C. (1975), 'Magnetic properties of Gd_2O_3', *Phys. Rev. B*, 11: 1609–22.
16. Blanusa, J., Antic, B., Kremenovic, A., Nikolic, A.S., Mazzerolles, L. et al. (2007), 'Particle size effect on Néel temperature in Er_2O_3 nanopowder synthesized by thermolysis of 2,4-pentadione complex', *Solid State Commun.*, 144: 310–14.
17. Xu, W., Kattel, K., Park, J.Y., Chang, Y., Kim, T.J. and Lee, G.H. (2012), 'Paramagnetic nanoparticle T_1 and T_2 MRI contrast agents', *Phys. Chem. Chem. Phys.*, 14: 12687–700.
18. Riss, T.L. and Moravec, R.A. (2004), 'Use of multiple assay endpoints to investigate the effects of incubation time, dose of toxin, and planting density in cell-based cytotoxicity assays', *Assay Drug Dev. Technol.*, 2: 51–62.
19. Decker, T. and Lohmann-Matthes, M.-L. (1988), 'A quick and simple method for the quantification of lactate dehydrogenase release in measurements of cellular cytotoxicity and tumor necrosis factor (TNF) activity', *J. Immunol. Methods*, 115: 61–9.

20. Borenfreund, E. and Puerner, J.A. (1984), 'A simple quantitative procedure using monolayer cultures for cytotoxicity assays (HTD/NR-90)', *J. Tissue Cul. Methods*, 9: 7–9.
21. Xu, W., Park, J.Y., Kattel, K., Bony, B.A., Heo, W.C. et al. (2012), 'A T_1, T_2 magnetic resonance imaging (MRI)-fluorescent imaging (FI) by using ultrasmall mixed gadolinium-europium oxide nanoparticles', *New J. Chem.*, 36: 2361–7.
22. Xu, W., Park, J.Y., Kattel, K., Ahmad, M.W., Bony, B.A, et al. (2012), 'Fluorescein-polyethyleneimine coated gadolinium oxide nanoparticles as T_1 magnetic resonance imaging (MRI)-cell labeling (CL) dual agents', *RSC Adv.*, 2: 10907–15.
23. Bünzli, J.-C.G. (2010), 'Lanthanide luminescence for biomedical analyses and imaging', *Chem. Rev.*, 110: 2729–55.
24. Eliseeva, S.V. and Bünzli, J.-C.G. (2010), 'Lanthanide luminescence for functional materials and bio-sciences', *Chem. Soc. Rev.*, 39: 1–380.
25. Wakefield, G., Keron, H.A., Dobson, P.J. and Hutchison, J.L. (1999), 'Synthesis and properties of sub-50-nm europium oxide nanoparticles', *J. Colloid Interface Sci.*, 215: 179–82.
26. Goldburt, E.T., Kulkarni, B., Bhargava, R.N., Taylor, J. and Libera, M. (1997), 'Size dependent efficiency in Tb doped Y_2O_3 nanocrystalline phosphor', *J. Lumin.*, 72–4: 190–2.

5

MRI, CT, FI, and multi-modal imaging and images

DOI: 10.1533/9780081000663.69

Abstract: This chapter discusses *in vivo* and *in vitro* application of ultrasmall lanthanide oxide nanoparticles to MRI, CT, FI, and multi-modal imaging. For each case, a simple theory of operation and one representative image is provided. To obtain MRI and CT images, a mouse is intravenously injected with an aqueous sample solution of biocompatible ligand coated ultrasmall lanthanide oxide nanoparticles and then *in vivo* images are obtained. To obtain *in vitro* FI images, biocompatible ligand coated ultrasmall lanthanide oxide nanoparticles are treated into cells, which are then incubated before *in vitro* cellular fluorescent confocal images are obtained. To obtain *in vivo* FI images, a small worm is fed with biocompatible ligand coated ultrasmall lanthanide oxide nanoparticles and *in vivo* fluorescent confocal images are obtained.

Key words: *in vivo, in vitro*, MRI, CT, FI, multi-modal imaging.

5.1 Magnetic resonance imaging (MRI) and images

A clinical MRI scanner is generally operated at 1.5 and 3.0 tesla magnetic fields. A 1.5 tesla MRI scanner is shown in Figure 5.1. In the case of a 1.5 tesla MRI scanner, a permanent magnet is generally used, whereas a superconducting electromagnet is used in a 3 tesla MRI scanner. A 7 tesla MRI scanner is not clinically used for humans, as it has not been proved to be safe, but is available for animal research. As the magnetic field increases, the energy splitting between α and β proton spins increases and therefore resolution of the image improves, because local protons can be more differentiated from one another at a higher magnetic field.

MRI images are generally obtained by applying a radiofrequency pulse. When a magnetic field is applied, a population difference between α and β spin states is produced, following Boltzmann distribution. A radiofrequency pulse is then applied and protons at a lower energy α spin (= 1/2) state become promoted to a higher energy β spin (= −1/2) state. When the radiofrequency pulse is stopped, relaxation of proton spins from high to low energy spin states can occur, producing a proton signal. Protons at different locations have different relaxation rates. These different rates, as well as different local proton densities, produce a MR image.

There are two types of MR images. One is a T_2 MR image that is obtained by recording transverse (T_2) relaxation of protons (*x*-*y* component of proton spin vector). The other is a T_1 MR image that is obtained by recording longitudinal (T_1) relaxation of protons (*z*-component of proton spin vector). Signal intensity (I) is given by [1]

$$I = e^{\frac{TE}{T_2}}\left(1 - e^{\frac{TR}{T_1}}\right) \qquad [5.1]$$

where TE is the time to echo, TR is the repetition time, T_1 is the longitudinal relaxation time, and T_2 is the transverse relaxation time.

In the presence of a T_1 contrast agent, such as ultrasmall gadolinium oxide nanoparticle, T_1 becomes shorter and thus the signal intensity (I) increases, making MR images brighter. On the other hand, in the presence of a T_2 MRI contrast agent, such as ultrasmall dysprosium oxide nanoparticle, T_2 becomes shorter and thus the signal intensity (I) decreases, making MR images darker. Theoretically, $r_2 \geq r_1$, in which r_1 is a longitudinal water proton relaxivity and r_2 is a transverse water proton relaxivity. Therefore, the r_1 value should be as large as possible and the r_2/r_1 ratio should be as close as possible to one for a T_1 MRI contrast agent, whereas both r_2 and r_2/r_1 ratio should be as large as possible for a T_2 MRI contrast agent. Here, the water proton relaxivity of a MRI contrast agent is defined by the number of protons relaxed per second and per unit mM Ln (Ln = lanthanide metal) of a MRI contrast agent. Thus, it has a unit of $s^{-1}mM^{-1}$.

Due to the variety of magnetic properties of lanthanide ions mentioned before, ultrasmall lanthanide oxide nanoparticles can be used as T_1 and/or T_2 MRI contrast agents, depending on the lanthanide ion. Ultrasmall gadolinium oxide nanoparticle is a potential T_1 MRI contrast agent, because of Gd(III) with spins (s) = 7/2. On the other hand, ultrasmall dysprosium oxide, holmium oxide, erbium oxide, and terbium oxide nanoparticles are potential T_2 MRI contrast agents at high MR fields, because of large magnetic moments of Dy(III) (10.4–10.6 μ_B), Ho(III) (10.4–10.7 μ_B), Er(III) (9.4–9.6 μ_B), and Tb(III) (9.5–9.8 μ_B) [2].

T_1 relaxation is accelerated by the interaction between a water proton with a β spin and a pure spin magnetic moment of metal ions of a MRI contrast agent. In the periodic table, Gd(III) has the largest s = 7/2 (7 unpaired 4f-electrons), and both Fe(III) and Mn(II) have the next largest $s = 5/2$ (5 unpaired 3d-electrons). Therefore, nanoparticles made of these metal ions can efficiently induce T_1 relaxation. This is because a slow electron spin motion is closely in tune with a slow proton spin relaxation. However, the electron orbital motion is so fast that it is far away from proton spin relaxation. Therefore, nanoparticles made of metal ions with electron orbital magnetic moment are not suitable as a T_1 MRI contrast agent. The r_1 value of gadolinium oxide nanoparticle is larger than that of Gd(III)-chelates, because of a dense population of Gd(III) in a nanoparticle. Gd(III)-chelates typically have a r_1 value ranging from 3 to 5 $s^{-1}mM^{-1}$, whereas gadolinium oxide nanoparticle has a r_1 value ranging from 10 to 15 $s^{-1}mM^{-1}$ [3].

However, T_2 relaxation is accelerated by a fluctuating local magnetic field produced by a nanoparticle. Therefore, a T_2 MRI contrast agent should have a large total magnetic moment at room temperature. The r_2 value is proportional to the square of a total magnetic moment of a MRI contrast agent. Therefore, a T_2 MRI contrast agent can be made only by nanoparticles and not by molecules. Some lanthanide elements such as Dy, Ho, Tb, and Er have large magnetic moments and so their oxide nanoparticles are potential T_2 MRI contrast agents. Recently, this was demonstrated, because several ultrasmall lanthanide oxide nanoparticles (d_{avg} <3 nm) had shown appreciable r_2 values [4]. Furthermore, an *in vivo* experiment in a mouse had shown clear T_2 contrast enhancements in liver and kidneys [4].

Nanoparticle MRI contrast agents have several advantages over molecular contrast agents. First, nanoparticles can circulate in a blood vessel longer than molecules and thus are suitable for blood-pool imaging agents. This also provides more chances for nanoparticles to be delivered into the region of interest, boosting imaging sensitivity. Second, when conjugated with drug and targeting agents, they can be used for diagnosis and therapy (the so-called theragnostic agent). However, nanoparticles should be smaller than 3 nm for renal excretion [5], because lanthanide oxide nanoparticles are generally toxic as there is no metabolic process to digest them in the body. This is different from iron oxide nanoparticles that can be digested in the body, because iron is an essential element in the body. The renal excretion can be monitored by taking MR images of kidneys and bladder as a function of time [6,7].

In vivo MR images are obtained after injecting an aqueous sample solution into a mouse tail vein. About 0.05 mmol Ln/kg is generally injected and MR images are taken as a function of time. After intravenous injection, contrast changes should be observed. That is, positive (or whiter) contrast enhancements are observed in the case of a T_1

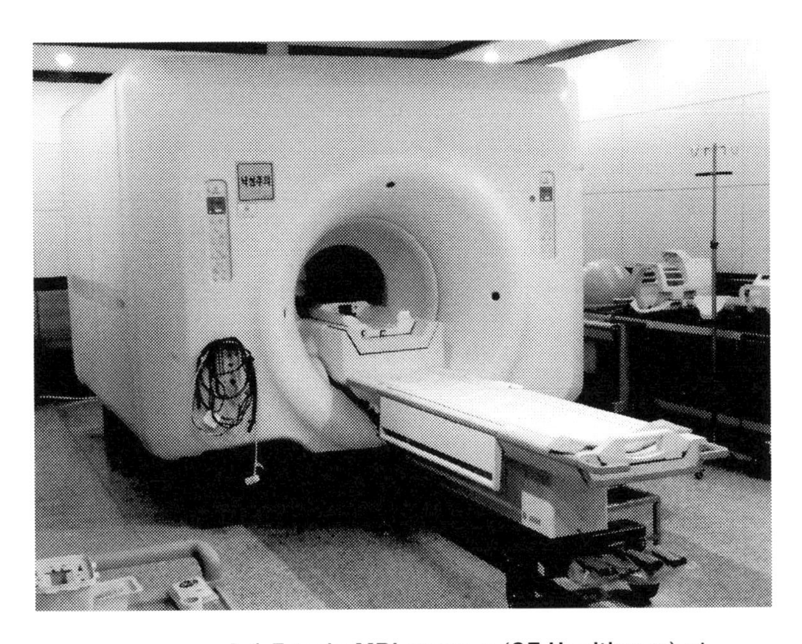

Figure 5.1 A 1.5 tesla MRI scanner (GE Healthcare) at Kyungpook National University Hospital, Taegu, South Korea

MRI contrast agent, whereas negative (or darker) contrast enhancements are observed in the case of a T_2 MRI contrast agent. Figure 5.2 shows T_1 MR images of a mouse taken after injection of an aqueous sample solution of D-glucuronic acid coated gadolinium oxide nanoparticles into a mouse tail vein. Clear positive (or whiter) contrast enhancements in T_1 MR images after intravenous injection can be seen at a brain tumor. MRI contrast agents tend to accumulate more into cancerous tissue than normal tissue, likely due to angiogenesis, Thus, cancer can be

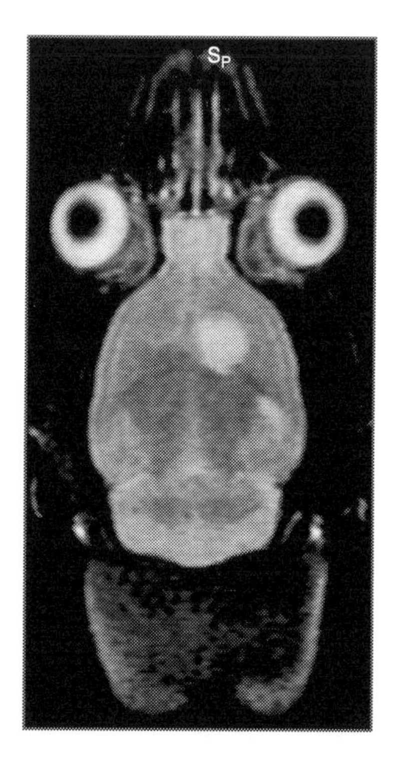

Figure 5.2 A T_1 MR image of a mouse taken after injection of an aqueous sample solution of D-glucuronic acid coated gadolinium oxide nanoparticles into a mouse tail vein (an arrow indicates a brain tumor)

detected through a contrast enhancement with respect to normal tissue.

5.2 X-ray computed tomography (CT) and images

The CT generates 2- and 3-dimensional images of the body. A schematic picture of a CT scanner is provided in Figure 5.3. To obtain a CT image slice, the X-ray source and X-ray detector rotate around a patient during the scan. The X-ray detector is located at the opposite side of the X-ray source. From each scan around the body, a 2-D slice image is obtained through sophisticated computation. A series of slice images are obtained moving both X-ray source and detector along the axis of a patient. A 3-D image is constructed by stacking all slice images. Since the X-ray is used as a radiation source, the CT is useful for imaging hard parts such as bones and hardened diseases in the body. However,

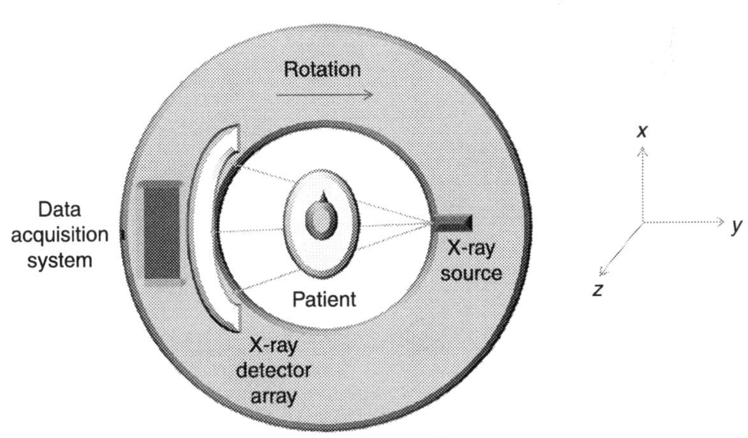

Figure 5.3 A schematic theory of operation of a CT scanner

with CT contrast agents, soft tissues such as blood vessels, heart, and muscles can be very sensitively imaged at a high resolution somewhat comparable to MRI.

Lanthanide elements have a higher X-ray attenuation power than iodine [8]. Therefore, ultrasmall lanthanide oxide nanoparticles can be a powerful CT contrast agent. Furthermore, ultrasmall lanthanide oxide nanoparticles are also useful for MRI contrast agents, implying that they are potential MRI-CT dual contrast agents. As a demonstration, *in vitro* phantom images of an aqueous sample solution of D-glucuronic acid coated gadolinium iodate ($Gd(IO_3)_3.2H_2O$) nanoparticles are provided in Figure 5.4. The figure clearly

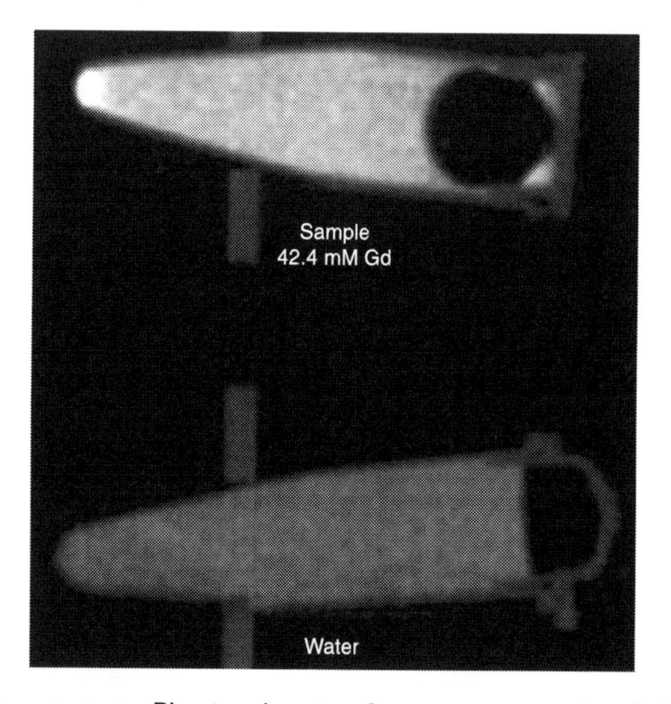

Figure 5.4 Phantom images of an aqueous sample solution of D-glucuronic acid coated gadolinium iodate ($Gd(IO_3)_3.2H_2O$) nanoparticles (top) and three-times distilled water as a reference (bottom)

shows contrast in a phantom image with respect to three-times distilled water.

5.3 Fluorescent imaging (FI) and images

Some lanthanide elements have strong fluorescence in the visible region [9,10]. For example, Eu and Tb fluoresce in the red and green regions, respectively. Therefore, these ultrasmall oxide nanoparticles can be used as a fluorescent imaging (FI) agent. FI agents should be strongly fluorescent and stable for a long time. Ultrasmall lanthanide oxide nanoparticles show an appreciable fluorescent intensity and their photostability is excellent, like quantum dots (QDs), because they are solid-state.

An imaging depth of FI is limited to a few millimeters, which is a disadvantage over other imaging modalities. However, by using an up-conversion composition, the imaging depth can be improved by up to a few centimeters. It is also found that fluorescent intensity of lanthanide oxide nanoparticles could increase with decreasing particle diameters [11,12], which will be beneficial for biomedical applications, because only ultrasmall nanoparticles can be excreted from the body through the renal system [5].

By doping Eu or Tb into ultrasmall gadolinium oxide or dysprosium oxide nanoparticles, mixed ultrasmall Gd/Eu, Gd/Tb, Dy/Eu, and Dy/Tb oxide nanoparticles can be used as a dual MRI-FI agent. These mixed nanoparticles have an advantage over core-shell, hetero-junction, and dye-coated nanoparticles, because of their compactness, robustness, stability, and easy synthesis with composition control [13].

A confocal laser scanning microscope equipped with a solid state laser can be used to record intracellular fluorescent images of cells and *in vivo* fluorescent images of small animals such as worms and insects [14]. *In vitro* cellular images can be taken by the following procedure. The cells are seeded onto two 35 mm cell culture dishes at a density of 2.5×10^5 (2 mL per dish, 5% CO_2, 37 °C). After 24 hours, one dish is treated with ~50 μL of an aqueous sample solution (40 mM Eu) and incubated for 48 hours. The treated cells are washed twice with a phosphate buffer saline (PBS) solution. The untreated cells in the other dish serve as a control cell. The cells in both dishes are fixed with 4% paraformaldehyde (PFA) in PBS solution for 10 minutes at room temperature and rewashed with PBS solution three times. The cell nuclei in both dishes are counterstained with 4′,6 diamidino-2-phenylindole (DAPI) and then rewashed with PBS solution three times. The cells are finally mounted using Prolong Gold (Invitrogen, Carlsbad, CA, USA) for imaging. One example is shown in Figure 5.5.

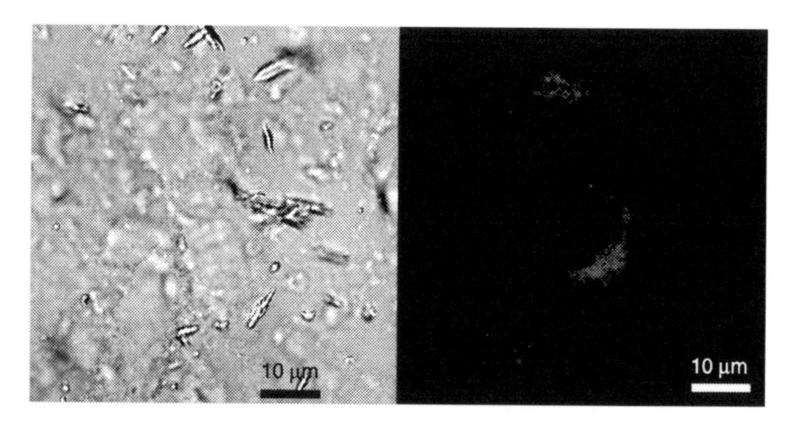

Figure 5.5 A fluorescent confocal image of DU145 cells incubated with D-glucuronic acid coated ultrasmall Eu_2O_3 nanoparticles before (left) and after (right) after excitation with 488 nm laser

The blue cell nuclei in the left figure are due to counterstaining with DAPI. Under these conditions, ~10^9 nanoparticles per cell with particle diameter of 1 to 3 nm can be internalized. The observed red fluorescence in the right figure is due to Eu(III) in nanoparticles.

In vivo images can be also obtained using a confocal laser scanning microscope. Since the imaging depth of FI is less than a few millimeters, only a small animal can be imaged. One example is the nematode, *C. elegans*, which is a N2 wild type worm [14]. For imaging purposes, they are prepared on a nematode growth medium (NGM)-agar dish at 22 °C. A 40 mM nanoparticle solution is made by dispersing a nanoparticle sample in 300 μL of NGM buffer (50 mM NaCl, 1 mM $CaCl_2$, 1 mM $MgSO_4$, and 25 mM K_3PO_4 in three-times distilled water) containing *Escherichia coli (E. coli)* strain OP50. This solution is sonicated for 10 minutes, pipetted onto a NGM-agar dish, and dried in air as food for *C. elegans. C. elegans* are starved for 48 hours and then transferred onto a NGM-agar dish using a pipette. They are left for 4 hours to feed. Some of the fed *C. elegans* are transferred onto an agar bed using a pipette and then sandwiched between two glass slips. *C. elegans* are fixed by adding a few drops of sodium azide solution (30 mM) for confocal imaging. Red fluorescence can be observed from ultrasmall Eu_2O_3 nanoparticles that are accumulated in the digestive system of *C. elegans* after laser excitation using 488 nm (Figure 5.6).

5.4 Multi-modal imaging

Lanthanide elements have a variety of magnetic and optical properties, depending on the lanthanide element [2,3]. Gd, Dy, Ho, Tb, and Er oxide nanoparticles with appreciable

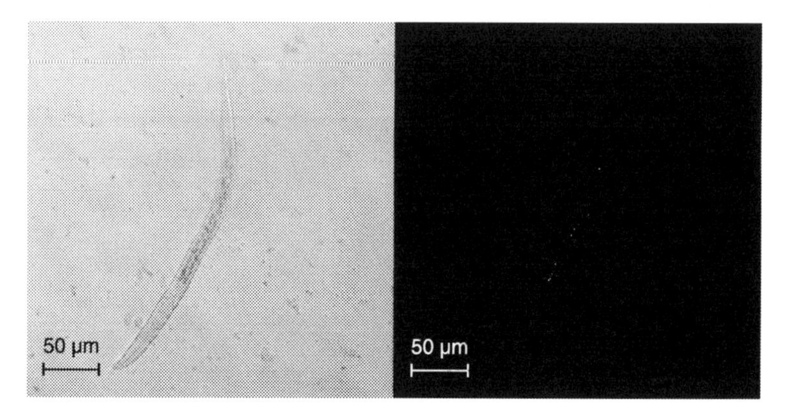

Figure 5.6 A fluorescent confocal image of intestines of a *C. elegans* after fed with D-glucuronic acid coated ultrasmall Eu_2O_3 nanoparticles: before (left) and after (right) excitation with 488 nm laser

magnetic moments at room temperature may be used for T_1 and/or T_2 MRI contrast agents. On the other hand, Eu and Tb oxide nanoparticles can be used as a FI agent, because they strongly fluoresce in the red (600 nm) and green (545 nm) regions, respectively. Ultrasmall lanthanide oxide nanoparticles also have high X-ray attenuation properties, so that they can be used as a CT contrast agent. Therefore, ultrasmall mixed or unmixed lanthanide oxide nanoparticles may be used for a multiple imaging agent such as a MRI-CT, a MRI-FI, or a CT-FI agent.

Ultrasmall mixed lanthanide oxide nanoparticles can be synthesized by mixing two different lanthanide precursors in solution. Owing to similar ionic radii, the common trivalent ionic state, similar reaction properties between lanthanide ions, and composition control in mixed lanthanide oxide nanoparticles can be easily done by simply varying a mole ratio of precursor ions. A variety of combination will also be possible, which include Gd/Eu, Dy/Eu, Ho/Tb, and Gd/Tb.

For example, MRI-FI dual imaging had been demonstrated using D-glucuronic acid coated ultrasmall Gd/Eu oxide nanoparticles [15]. MRI was demonstrated by taking T_1 and T_2 MR images before and after intravenous injection of an aqueous sample solution into a mouse tail vein, while FI was demonstrated by taking cellular confocal images after incubating ultrasmall Gd/Eu nanoparticles into DU145 cells. Obtained MR and FI images are similar to those given in Figures 5.2 and 5.5, respectively.

Multimodal imaging of ultrasmall lanthanide oxide nanoparticles can be extended by conjugating a variety of other imaging agents. For example, by conjugating dye to them, MRI-FI or CT-FI will be possible. One example is fluorescein conjugated Gd_2O_3 nanoparticles, in which fluorescein strongly fluoresces in the green region (496 nm), while Gd_2O_3 nanoparticles function as a T_1 MRI contrast agent [16].

5.5 References

1. Hashemi, R.H., Bradley, W.G. and Lisanti, C.J. (2004), *MRI The Basics*, 2nd edn, New York: Lippincott Williams & Wilkins.
2. Greenwood, N.N. and Earnshaw, A. (1997), *Chemistry of the Elements*, Oxford, UK: Butterworth-Heinemann, 2nd edn, p. 1243.
3. Kim, T.J., Chae, K.S., Chang, Y. and Lee, G.H. (2013), 'Gadolinium oxide nanoparticles as potential multimodal imaging and therapeutic agents', *Curr. Topics Med. Chem.*, 13: 422–33.
4. Kattel, K., Park, J.Y., Xu, W., Kim, H.G., Lee, E.J. et al. (2011), 'A facile synthesis, *in vitro* and *in vivo* MR studies of D-glucuronic acid-coated ultrasmall Ln_2O_3

(Ln = Eu, Gd, Dy, Ho, and Er) nanoparticles as a new potential MRI contrast agent', *ACS Appl. Mater. Interfaces*, 3: 3325–34.

5. Choi, H.S., Liu, W., Misra, P., Tanaka, E., Zimmer, J.P. et al. (2007), 'Renal clearance of quantum dots', *Nat. Biotechnology*, 25: 1165–70.
6. Park, J.Y., Baek, M.J., Choi, E.S., Woo, S., Kim, J.H. et al. (2009), 'Paramagnetic ultrasmall gadolinium oxide nanoparticles as advanced T_1 MRI contrast agent: account for large longitudinal relaxivity, optimal particle diameter, and *in vivo* T_1 MR images', *ACS Nano*, 3: 3663–9.
7. Bridot, J.-L., Faure, A.-C., Laurent, S., Rivière, C., Billotey, C. et al. (2007), 'Hybrid gadolinium oxide nanoparticles: multimodal contrast agents for *in vivo* imaging', *J. Am. Chem. Soc.*, 129: 5076–84.
8. Hubbell, J.H. and Seltzer, S.M. (1995), 'Tables of X-ray mass attenuation coefficients and mass energy-absorption coefficients from 1 keV to 20 MeV for elements Z = 1 to 92 and 48 additional substances of dosimetric interest', NIST Technical Report (PB-95-220539/XAB).
9. Bünzli, J.-C.G. (2010), 'Lanthanide luminescence for biomedical analyses and imaging', *Chem. Rev.*, 110: 2729–55.
10. Eliseeva, S.V. and Bünzli, J.-C.G. (2010), 'Lanthanide luminescence for functional materials and bio-sciences', *Chem. Soc. Rev.*, 39: 1–380.
11. Wakefield, G., Keron, H.A., Dobson, P.J. and Hutchison, J.L. (1999), 'Synthesis and properties of sub-50-nm europium oxide nanoparticles', *J. Colloid Interface Sci.*, 215: 179–82.
12. Goldburt, E.T., Kulkarni, B., Bhargava, R.N., Taylor, J. and Libera, M. (1997), 'Size dependent efficiency in

Tb doped Y_2O_3 nanocrystalline phosphor', *J. Lumin.*, 72–4: 190–2.

13. Xu, W., Bony, B.A., Kim, C.R., Baeck, J.S., Chang, Y. et al. (2013), 'Mixed lanthanide oxide nanoparticles as dual imaging agent in biomedicine', *Scientific Reports* 3: 3210 (published on-line 13 November 2013).
14. Kattel, K., Park, J.Y., Xu, W., Kim, H.G., Lee, E.J. et al. (2012), 'Water-soluble ultrasmall Eu_2O_3 nanoparticles as a fluorescent imaging agent: *in vitro* and *in vivo* studies', *Colloids. Surf. A: Physicochem. Eng. Aspects*, 394: 85–91.
15. Xu, W., Park, J.Y., Kattel, K., Bony, B.A., Heo, W.C. et al. (2012), 'A T_1, T_2 magnetic resonance imaging (MRI)-fluorescent imaging (FI) by using ultrasmall mixed gadolinium-europium oxide nanoparticles', *New J. Chem.*, 36: 2361–7.
16. Xu, W., Park, J.Y., Kattel, K., Ahmad, M.W., Bony, B.A. et al. (2012), 'Fluorescein-polyethyleneimine coated gadolinium oxide nanoparticles as T_1 magnetic resonance imaging (MRI)-cell labeling (CL) dual agents', *RSC Adv.*, 2: 10907–15.

6

A simple model calculation of water proton relaxivities

DOI: 10.1533/9780081000663.85

Abstract: This chapter discusses a simple model calculation of longitudinal (r_1) and transverse (r_2) water proton relaxivities of ultrasmall lanthanide oxide nanoparticles. The model assumes an induction mechanism of longitudinal (T_1) and transverse (T_2) water proton relaxations by paramagnetic nanoparticles. The model broadly accounts for r_1 and r_2 values. Calculated r_1 and r_2 values are compared with experimental values.

Key words: simple model calculation, water proton relaxivity, paramagnetic nanoparticle.

6.1 Introduction

This chapter deals with ultrasmall lanthanide (Ln) oxide nanoparticles (Ln = Gd, Dy, Tb, Ho, and Er) that can be used as MRI contrast agents [1]. They can also be used as a CT contrast agent, a FI agent, a multimodal imaging agent, and a NCT theragnostic agent, depending on the nanoparticle species, as discussed in the previous chapters [2]. They are paramagnetic and therefore their magnetizations are not fully saturated at room temperature [1,2]. However, they show decent magnetizations at room temperature, because of large magnetic moments of the lanthanides [3], and even at ultrasmall particle diameters, because their magnetizations are nearly insensitive to particle diameter and surface conditions. Their saturation magnetizations that can be obtained at low temperatures are very large and much larger than that of iron oxide nanoparticles [1]. These decent magnetic moments at room temperature make them strongly induce longitudinal (T_1) and/or transverse (T_2) water proton relaxations, depending on the nanoparticle species.

Theories on water proton relaxivities have been developed on metal-chelates [4,5] and superparamagnetic nanoparticles [6–8]. These theories are very complex to use and might not be suitable for paramagnetic nanoparticles. Therefore, a very simple and empirical model to calculate longitudinal (r_1) and transverse (r_2) water proton relaxivities of paramagnetic nanoparticle is provided in this chapter. The model broadly assumes T_1 and T_2 water proton relaxations induced by a paramagnetic nanoparticle. The r_1 and r_2 values are calculated using the model and compared with experimental values.

6.2 Magnetization

An ultrasmall lanthanide oxide (Ln_2O_3) nanoparticle is paramagnetic. Therefore, the metal ion spins in a nanoparticle are independent. In the absence of an external field (H), the net magnetic moment is zero at room temperature, because spins are random (Figure 6.1(a)). In the presence of H, the metal ion spins somewhat align along the H, producing a decent net magnetic moment (M_{NP}) at room temperature (Figure 6.1(b)). The magnitude of the net magnetic moment

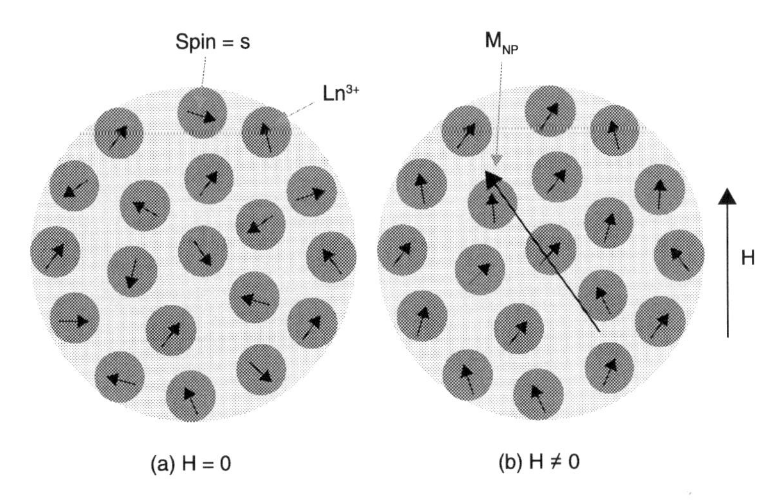

Figure 6.1 Schematic diagrams of the spin structure of an ultrasmall Ln_2O_3 nanoparticle: (a) external field (H) is off and (b) H is on

of a Ln_2O_3 nanoparticle depends on Ln. It is high for Ln = Gd, Tb, Dy, Ho, and Er, because these Ln have large magnetic moments [3]. Therefore, ultrasmall lanthanide oxide nanoparticles made of these Ln are potential MRI contrast agents [1].

Magnetization at clinical temperature (i.e. T = 37 °C) and at clinical applied fields (i.e. H = 1.5 and 3.0 tesla) is important for MRI. To investigate the magnetization of ultrasmall lanthanide oxide nanoparticles under these conditions, magnetization versus applied field curves (i.e. M-H curves) of ultrasmall Ln_2O_3 (Ln = Eu, Gd, Dy, Ho, Er) nanoparticles are shown in Figure 6.2. The figure shows that magnetization is linear with respect to H. Therefore, M-H curves can be fit to a linear function of $M = aH + b$, to obtain M at any H of interest. The fitted equations and magnetizations at H = 1.5, 3.0, and 5 tesla are shown in Table 6.1.

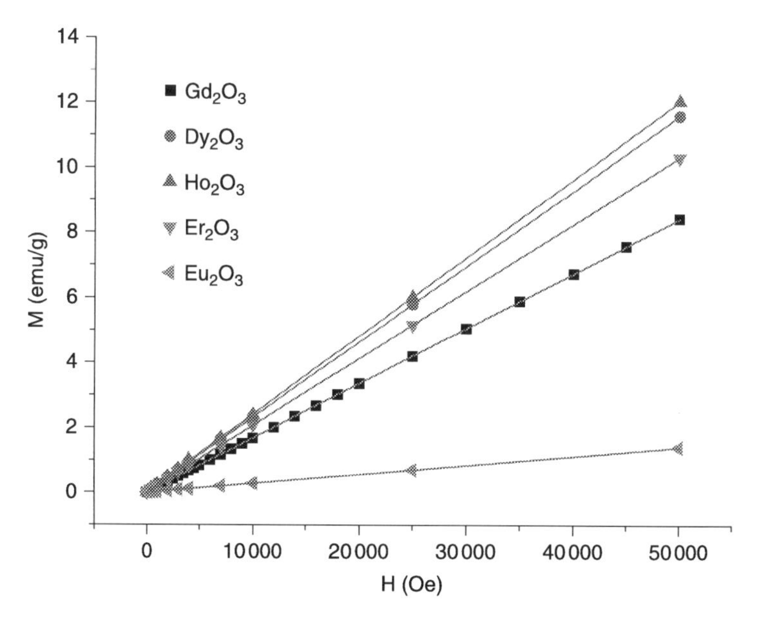

Figure 6.2 Plots of M-H curves for ultrasmall Ln_2O_3 nanoparticles. Each curve is fit to a linear function of $M = aH + b$

Table 6.1 Magnetization of ultrasmall Ln_2O_3 nanoparticles ($Ln = Eu$, Gd, Dy, Ho, and Er)

Nano-particle	Fitted equation	Magnetization (emu/g) at three applied fields (tesla)		
		1.5	3.0	5.0
Eu_2O_3	$M = 2.8013 \times 10^{-5} H - 7.22784 \times 10^{-4}$	0.42	0.84	1.40
Gd_2O_3	$M = 1.68601 \times 10^{-4} H - 0.00956$	2.52	5.05	8.42
Dy_2O_3	$M = 2.31963 \times 10^{-4} H - 0.00262$	3.48	6.96	11.60
Ho_2O_3	$M = 2.40795 \times 10^{-4} H + 0.00183$	3.61	7.22	12.04
Er_2O_3	$M = 2.06264 \times 10^{-4} H + 0.00354$	3.10	6.19	10.32

6.3 Longitudinal water proton relaxation (T_1) and relaxivity (r_1)

In the absence of an external field (H), the energy of α and β spins of water protons degenerate (Figure 6.3(a)). When H is applied, the degenerated water proton energy is split into two states (Figure 6.3(b)). It is assumed that the distribution of water proton spins in these two states follows the Boltzmann distribution (Figure 6.3(c)). When a radiofrequency pulse is applied, the low energy state protons with α (= 1/2) spin become excited into a higher energy state with β (= −1/2) spin [9]. When a radiofrequency pulse stops, spins relax from β to α spins, emitting radiofrequency photons. Intensity of emitted photons depends on local protons, because the proton density and proton relaxation rate are local. This difference forms a MR image, with a spatial resolution of approximately 1 mm. In the presence of a MRI contrast agent, the relaxation rate is enhanced, enhancing signal intensities of local protons, which in turn makes local protons more differentiated from others (the so-called contrast enhancement), providing a higher spatial

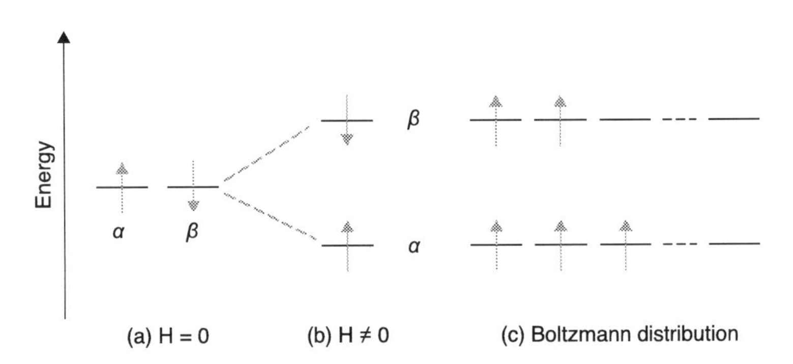

Figure 6.3 An energy splitting of water proton α and β spins in the presence of external field (H)

resolution MR image. For example, capillary vessels can be clearly distinguished.

T_1 relaxation is the relaxation of the *z*-component of a proton spin vector [9]. In the presence of a MRI contrast agent, T_1 relaxation is enhanced from the interaction between the proton β spin magnetic moment and the metal ion spin magnetic moment that is strong because a slow electron spin motion is closely matched with the slow proton spin relaxation. On the other hand, an electron orbital motion is so fast that the orbital magnetic moment contributes very little to inducing the proton relaxation from β to α spins. Among the lanthanides, only Gd^{3+} has a pure electron spin magnetic moment of $s=7/2$, because it has 7 unpaired 4f-electrons. Other Ln^{3+} ions have both orbital and spin components in their electron magnetic moment, therefore, they are not suitable for inducing T_1 relaxation. Both Fe^{3+} and Mn^{2+} also have a pure spin magnetic moment of $s=5/2$, because of their 5 unpaired 3d-electrons and thus they can also induce T_1 relaxation. Since nanoparticles are composed of numerous metal ions, they can more strongly induce T_1 relaxation than metal chelates.

A simple model describing the induction of T_1 relaxation by a paramagnetic nanoparticle is provided in Figure 6.4(a). An ultrasmall gadolinium oxide nanoparticle contains many Gd^{3+}. Therefore, it can more strongly induce T_1 relaxation than Gd-chelates [10]. As schematically drawn in Figure 6.4(a), the model proposes that T_1 relaxation of a high energy state with β spin (= −1/2) into a lower energy state with α spin (= 1/2) is induced by a pure spin magnetic moment (m_s) of individual metal ions in a nanoparticle. For simplicity, assuming that r_1 is mainly induced by metal ions in a nanoparticle close to the β spin of the proton, r_1 at a given metal ion concentration can be written as

$r_1 \propto Nm_s^{\ 2} \approx$ (spin magnetic moment of a metal ion, $m_s = \sqrt{s(s+1)})^2$ (metal ion number density in a nanoparticle) (surface to volume ratio of a nanoparticle)

$$\approx s(s+1)\left(\frac{\frac{\frac{4}{3}\pi R^3}{\frac{4}{3}\pi l^3}}{\frac{4}{3}\pi R^3}\right)\frac{4\pi R^2}{\frac{4}{3}\pi R^3} = \frac{s(s+1)}{Rl^3} \quad [6.1]$$

in which N is the number of Ln^{3+} in a nanoparticle close to the β spin of the proton that contributes to induction of T_1 relaxation of that proton (indicated with a dotted circle in Figure 6.4(a)), s is the metal ion spin magnetic moment quantum number, R is the nanoparticle radius, and l is the

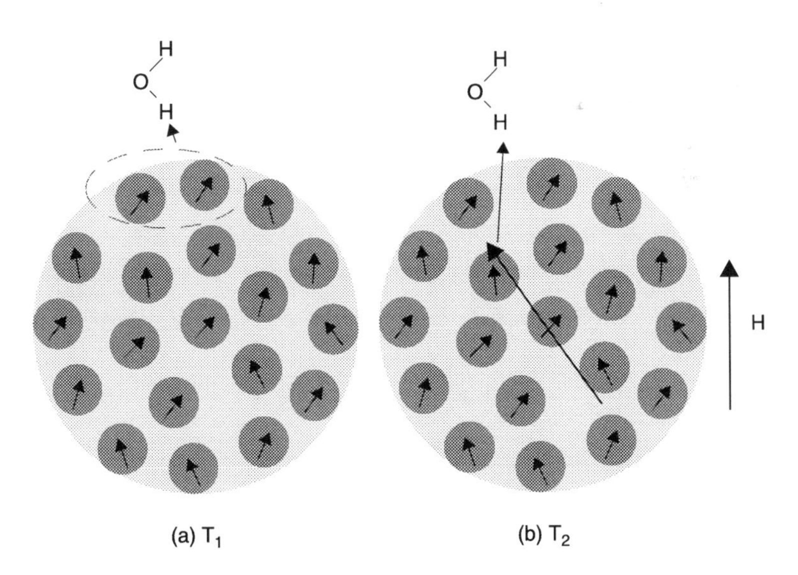

Figure 6.4 Schematic diagrams of a simple model: (a) T_1 relaxation; and (b) T_2 relaxation induced by a paramagnetic nanoparticle

metal ion radius at the coordination number of 6 [11]. Calculated r_1 values are scaled with respect to that of a Gd_2O_3 nanoparticle with $R = 1.2$ nm (Table 6.2). As can be seen from the table, the scaled r_1 values are fairly consistent with experimental values [12, 13] implying that this simple model accounts for the induction of T_1 relaxation by a paramagnetic nanoparticle.

6.4 Transverse water proton relaxation (T_2) and relaxivity (r_2)

T_2 relaxation is the relaxation of the *x*-*y*-component of a proton spin vector. As shown in Figure 6.4(b), it is induced by a fluctuation of a local magnetic field generated by a nanoparticle with a magnetic moment of M_{NP}. As R increases, M_{NP} increases, but the number of nanoparticles decrease at a given concentration. r_2 is proportional to the square of M_{NP}^2, the number of nanoparticles in a solution sample that is anti-proportional to the number of metal ions in a nanoparticle, and the number of water molecules around a nanoparticle surface that is proportional to the surface area of a nanoparticle. r_2 is also related to the distance between the proton β spin and M_{NP}. Assuming a point M_{NP} centered at a nanoparticle with $1/R^3$ dependence for the magnetic dipole interaction energy between M_{NP} and the water proton β spin, r_2 at a given metal ion concentration can be written as

$$r_2 \propto M_{NP}^2 \times (\text{number of nanoparticles}) \times (\text{number of water molecules around a nanoparticle}) \times (1/R^3)$$

$$\approx M_{NP}^2 \times (\text{number of water molecules around a nanoparticle})/\{(\text{number of metal ions in a nanoparticle}) \times R^3\}$$

Table 6.2 Calculated r_1 and r_2 values at 1.5 tesla

Nanoparticle	R (nm)	s	l (nm)	M (emu/g)	$M_{NP} \times 10^{-19}$ (emu/nanoparticle)	Experimental		Calculated and Scaled	
						r_1 ($mM^{-1}s^{-1}$)	r_2 ($mM^{-1}s^{-1}$)	r_1 ($mM^{-1}s^{-1}$)	r_2 ($mM^{-1}s^{-1}$)
Eu_2O_3	1.0	0	0.0947	0.42	1.30	0.006 [1]	3.82 [1]	0.0	0.54 (0.65)
Gd_2O_3	0.5	7/2	0.0938	2.52	0.98	9.9 [12]	10.5 [12]	10.20	4.70 (11.30)
Gd_2O_3	1.2	7/2	0.0938	2.52	13.51	4.25 [1]	27.11 [1]	4.25	27.11 (27.11)
Dy_2O_3	1.45	0	0.0912	3.48	34.71	0.16 [1]	40.28 [1]	0.0	77.10 (63.80)
Dy_2O_3	1.6	0	0.0912	3.48	46.58	0.008 [13]	65.04 [13]	0.0	93.70 (70.30)
Ho_2O_3	1.2	0	0.0901	3.61	21.87	0.13 [1]	31.24 [1]	0.0	63.00 (62.97)
Er_2O_3	1.45	0	0.0890	3.10	34.18	0.06 [1]	14.74 [1]	0.0	69.50 (57.50)

$$\approx \frac{\left[M\rho\left(\frac{4}{3}\pi R^3\right)\right]^2}{\dfrac{\frac{4}{3}\pi R^3}{\frac{4}{3}\pi l^3}} \times 4\pi R^2 \times \frac{1}{R^3} = \frac{64}{9}\pi^3 M^2 \rho^2 R^2 l^3 \qquad [6.2]$$

in which M is the magnetization estimated from M-H curves at 1.5 tesla and 300 K and ρ is the bulk density of a nanoparticle [14]. M_{NP} was roughly estimated by multiplying M with a mass of a nanoparticle that is obtained by multiplying ρ with a volume of a nanoparticle (Equation 6.2). Calculated r_2 values are scaled with respect to that of a Gd_2O_3 nanoparticle with R = 1.2 nm (Table 6.2). Scaled r_2 values are roughly consistent with experimental values. If the magnetic dipole interaction force (i.e. $1/R^4$) between M_{NP} and the water proton β spin is used instead of the magnetic dipole interaction energy (i.e. $1/R^3$), scaled r_2 values (given in parentheses) are for some reason more consistent with experimental values.

6.5 Concluding remarks

A simple theory is suggested to estimate r_1 and r_2 values of paramagnetic nanoparticles. This theory is applied to ultrasmall lanthanide oxide nanoparticles and the results are fairly satisfactory. Therefore, it can be used to predict approximate r_1 and r_2 values of other paramagnetic nanoparticles.

6.6 References

1. Kattel, K., Park, J.Y., Xu, W., Kim, H.G., Lee, E.J. et al. (2011), 'A facile synthesis, *in vitro* and *in vivo* MR

studies of D-glucuronic acid-coated ultrasmall Ln_2O_3 (Ln = Eu, Gd, Dy, Ho, and Er) nanoparticles as a new potential MRI contrast agent', *ACS Appl. Mater. Interfaces*, 3: 3325–34.

2. Xu, W., Kattel, K., Park, J.Y., Chang, Y., Kim, T.J. and Lee, G.H. (2012), 'Paramagnetic nanoparticle T_1 and T_2 MRI contrast agents', *Phys. Chem. Chem. Phys.*, 14: 12687–700.
3. Greenwood, N.N. and Earnshaw, A. (1997), *Chemistry of the Elements*, 2nd edn, Oxford, UK: Butterworth-Heinemann, p. 1243.
4. Lauffer, R.B. (1987), 'Paramagnetic metal complexes as water proton relaxation agents for NMR imaging: theory and design', *Chem. Rev.*, 87: 901–27.
5. Caravan, P., Ellison, J.J., McMurry, T.J. and Lauffer, R.B. (1999), 'Gadolinium(III) chelates as MRI contrast agents: structure, dynamics, and applications', *Chem. Rev.*, 99: 2293–352.
6. Roch, A., Muller, R.N. and Gillis, P. (1999), 'Theory of proton relaxation induced by superparamagnetic particles', J. *Phys. Chem.*, 110: 5403–11.
7. Roch, A., Gossuin, Y., Muller, R.N. and Gillis, P. (2005), 'Superparamagnetic colloid suspensions: Water magnetic relaxation and clustering', *J. Magn. Magn. Mater.*, 293: 532–9.
8. Norek, M., Pereira, G.A., Geraldes, C.F.G.C., Denkova, A., Zhou, W. and Peters, J.A. (2007), *J. Phys. Chem.* C, 111: 10240–6.
9. Hashemi, R.H., Bradley, W.G. and Lisanti, C.J. (2004), *MRI The Basics*, 2nd edn, New York: Lippincott Williams & Wilkins.
10. Kim, T.J., Chae, K.S., Chang, Y. and Lee, G.H. (2013), 'Gadolinium oxide nanoparticles as potential

multimodal imaging and therapeutic agents', *Curr. Topics Med. Chem.*, 13: 422–33.

11. Dean, J.A. (1992), *Lange's Handbook of Chemistry*, New York: McGraw-Hill, pp. 4.14–4.15.
12. Park, J.Y., Baek, M.J., Choi, E.S., Woo, S., Kim, J.H. et al. (2009), 'Paramagnetic ultrasmall gadolinium oxide nanoparticles as advanced T_1 MRI contrast agent: account for large longitudinal relaxivity, optimal particle diameter, and *in vivo* T_1 MR images', *ACS Nano*, 3: 3663–9.
13. Kattel, K., Park, J.Y., Xu, W., Kim, H.G., Lee, E.J. et al. (2012), 'Paramagnetic dysprosium oxide nanoparticles and dysprosium hydroxide nanorods as T_2 MRI contrast agents', *Biomaterials*, 33: 3254–61.
14. Aldrich Catalog (2005/06), p. 1260 (Gd_2O_3), p. 1085 (Dy_2O_3), p. 1330 (Ho_2O_3), p. 1094 (Er_2O_3), and p. 1509 (MnO).

7

Thermal neutron capture therapy (NCT)

DOI: 10.1533/9780081000663.97

Abstract: ^{157}Gd has the largest neutron capture cross-section (of 257 000) barns among the stable radio isotopes, that is 67 times larger than that of ^{10}B. Therefore, ultrasmall gadolinium oxide nanoparticles are a potential neutron capture therapy (NCT) agent. Since ultrasmall gadolinium oxide nanoparticles can be also used as a MRI contrast agent, they can also be used as a MRI-NCT theragnostic agent.

Key words: ^{157}Gd, NCT, ultrasmall gadolinium oxide nanoparticle, theragnostic agent.

7.1 Introduction

Development of a new treatment technique of cancers is a challenging subject. One such technique is neutron capture therapy (NCT). NCT is an almost non-invasive technique, because it makes use of a low dose of thermal neutron (energy less than 0.1 eV.), which does not damage normal cells. NCT was begun with ^{10}B (so-called BNCT) by G.L. Locher at the Franklin Institute in Pennsylvania, USA. After his suggestion, many scientists began research in USA, Europe, and Asia.

The theory of operation of NCT is presented in Figure 7.1. Radio nuclides in a molecular form are exclusively targeted into cancer cells, absorb thermal neutrons, and emit α-particles, electrons, γ-rays, etc. The emitted α-particles and/or electrons break the cancer cells by damaging the DNA in cancer cell nuclei. The success of NCT entirely depends on the targeting ability of the chemicals. They should be exclusively targeted into cancer cells, avoiding damaging normal cells. Based on neutron capture cross-section, ^{157}Gd (natural abundance = 15.7%) is a very promising radionuclide,

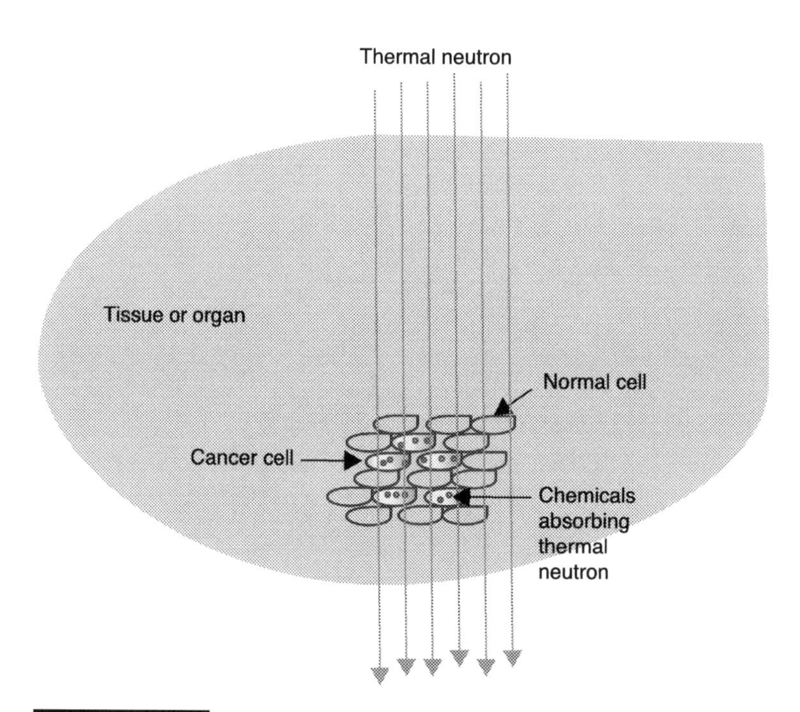

Figure 7.1 The theory of operation of NCT

because of its high neutron capture cross-section of 257 000 barns (1 barn = 10^{-24} m^2, the size of uranium nucleus), the highest among the stable radio-isotopes [1]. *In vitro* cell studies, as well as a few *in vivo* animal studies, have proved that the cancer cells targeted with ^{157}Gd-compounds were damaged after thermal neutron irradiation, showing the possibility of GdNCT [2–7].

The thermal neutron can be generated using either a nuclear reactor or a cyclotron accelerator. For clinical applications, a cyclotron accelerator is more useful because its costs are low, has a small-size, and can be easily installed at the hospital. A cyclotron accelerator is shown in Figure 7.2 (left). A patient is treated in the neutron beam irradiation facility room (Figure 7.2 (right)), which is isolated from the cyclotron accelerator by a heavy lead plate for safety. The thermal neutron beam is irradiated towards the cancer cell, being targeted through a small hole. The thermal neutron beam flux, energy, and diameter are the parameters to be optimized to obtain the best NCT.

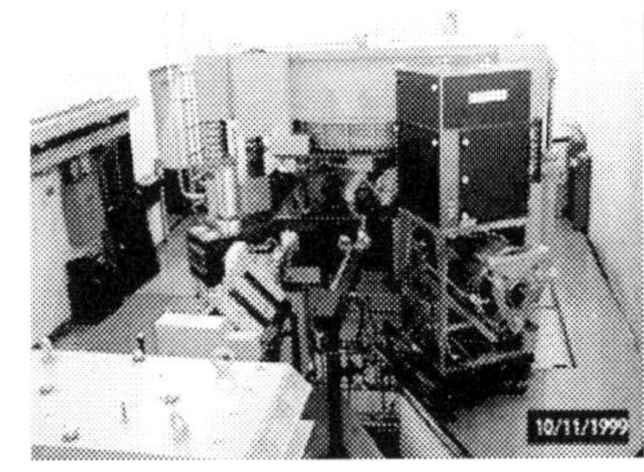

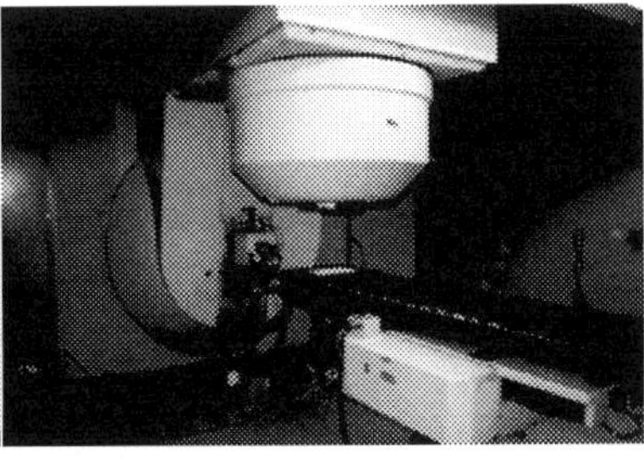

Figure 7.2 A cyclotron accelerator (left) that generates a thermal neutron and a neutron beam irradiation facility (right) at KIRMS, Seoul, South Korea

7.2 BNCT

^{10}B (natural abundance = 19.6%) has a thermal neutron capture cross-section of 3840 barns. After capturing a thermal neutron, ^{10}B becomes excited into ^{11}B, which generates ^{11}Li and an α-particle (Equation 7.1). Both ^{11}Li and α-particle can contribute to cancer cell damage by denaturing the double-helix of the DNA. Both ^{11}Li and α-particle have a penetration depth of less than 10 μm, corresponding to a cell diameter. Therefore, ^{10}B-chemicals should be close to or inside the cancer cell nuclei:

$$^{10}B + n_{thermal} \rightarrow [^{11}Li] \rightarrow \alpha(1.47\,MeV) + {}^{7}Li\ (0.84\,MeV) \qquad [7.1]$$

Two BNCT agents have been clinically used for patients. These include boronophenylalanine (BPA, $C_9H_{12}BNO_4$) and mercaptoundecahydrododecaborate-^{10}B or sodium borocaptate (BSH, $Na_2B_{12}H_{11}SH$) [8]. In addition, many B-chemicals are now under development.

7.3 GdNCT

GdNCT using ^{157}Gd is more powerful than BNCT using ^{10}B, because ^{157}Gd has a neutron capture cross-section 67 times larger as that of ^{10}B. ^{157}Gd captures a thermal neutron and becomes ^{158}Gd, which generates γ-rays and electrons as shown in the following [5]:

$$^{157}Gd + n_{thermal} \rightarrow {}^{158}Gd + \gamma(7.88\,MeV) + ACK - electrons\ (4.2\,keV) \qquad [7.2]$$

Among the reaction products, Auger and Coster-Kronig (ACK) electrons participate in cancer cell damage by indirectly damaging DNA in the cancer cell nuclei. ACK electrons react with water and then generate reactive OH^-, which denatures the double-helix DNA. Since electrons have a short penetration distance of less than 10 μm, corresponding to the cell diameter, Gd-chemicals should be close to or inside the cancer cell nuclei. The high energy γ-ray (7.88 MeV) is also effective in damaging cancer cells [6]. It has a long penetration depth of 10 cm or so. A theoretical simulation study showed that a 5 Gy (1 gray = 1 J/kg) is enough to damage cancer cells. However, it could also damage normal cells, because of its long penetration depth.

GdNCT studies using MRI contrast agents such as Gd-DTPA and Gd-DOTA have shown that GdNCT is effective in damaging cancer cells [3,5]. However, their targeting percentage to cancel cells was not high. Therefore, new Gd-chemicals with high targeting capabilities should be developed. Ultrasmall gadolinium oxide nanoparticles have been used for GdNCT *in vitro* in lymphoma cells (EL4-Luc), showing cancer damage after thermal neutron irradiation [7]. Ultrasmall gadolinium oxide nanoparticles will be much more powerful for GdNCT than molecular Gd-chemicals, because of the abundance of ^{157}Gd per nanoparticles.

In addition to a higher thermal neutron capture cross-section, GdNCT has an advantage over BNCT. GdNCT agents in the form of ultrasmall gadolinium oxide nanoparticles can be used as a T_1 MRI contrast agent. Therefore, GdNCT agents can be used for both cancer cell diagnosis and therapy. That is, after intravenous injection, the cancer cell can be first diagnosed with MRI and then treated with GdNCT. If GdNCT is commercialized, it will be a new and ideal theragnostic method to treat cancers.

7.4 References

1. Mughabghab, S.F. (2003), 'Thermal neutron capture cross-sections: resonance integrals and g-factors, IAEA Nuclear Data Section', Wagramer Strasse 5, A-1400, Vienna.
2. Mitin, V.N., Kulakov, V.N., Khokhlov, V.F., Sheino, I.N., Arnopolskaya, A.M. et al. (2009), 'Comparison of BNCT and GdNCT efficacy in treatment of canine cancer', *Appl. Radiation Isotopes*, 67: S299–S301.
3. De Stasio, G., Casalbore, P., Pallini, R., Gilbert, B., Sanita, F., et al. (2001), 'Gadolinium in human glioblastoma cells for gadolinium neutron capture therapy', *Cancer Res.*, 61: 4272–7.
4. Gierga, D.P., Yanch, J.C. and Shefer, R.E. (2000), 'An investigation of the feasibility of gadolinium for neutron capture synovectomy', *Med. Phys.*, 27: 1685–92.
5. De Stasio, G., Rajesh, D., Casalbore, P., Daniels, M.J., Erhardt, R.J. et al. (2005), 'Are gadolinium contrast agents suitable for gadolinium neutron capture therapy?' *Neurological Res.*, 27: 387–98.
6. Masiakowski, J.T., Horton, J.L. and Peters, L.J. (1992), 'Gadolinium neutron capture therapy for brain tumors: a computer study', *Med. Phys.*, 19: 1277–84.
7. Bridot, J.-L., Dayde, D., Riviere, C., Mandon, C., Billotey, C. et al. (2009), 'Hybrid gadolinium oxide nanoparticles combining imaging and therapy', *J. Mater. Chem.*, 19: 2328–35.
8. Barth, R.F., Coderre, J.A., Vicente, M.G.H. and Blue, T.E. (2005), 'Boron neutron capture therapy of cancer: current status and future prospects', *Clin. Cancer Res.*, 11: 3987–4002.

8

Perspectives and challenges

DOI: 10.1533/9780081000663.103

Abstract: Perspective and challenge of ultrasmall lanthanide oxide nanoparticles in nanomedicine are discussed. This summarizes possible application of ultrasmall lanthanide oxide nanoparticles to various imaging areas and therapy that are discussed in this book. In addition, this chapter briefly discusses what needs to be done for clinical applications.

Key words: perspective, challenge, ultrasmall lanthanide oxide nanoparticle.

8.1 Perspectives and challenges

Although many nanoparticle species have been investigated so far for biomecical applications, ultrasmall lanthanide oxide nanoparticles seem to be the most versatile ones. Therefore, they are the promising materials in diagnosis and treatment in biomedicine. Their diverse applications arise from a variety of magnetic and optical properties of lanthanide elements. Owing to these diverse properties, ultrasmall lanthanide oxide and mixed lanthanide oxide nanoparticles can be applied to a variety of single and multimodal imaging. In addition, ^{157}Gd has a very large thermal neutron capture cross-section. Therefore, Gd-containing nanoparticles can be applied to neutron capture therapy (NCT) (so-called GdNCT), as well as MRI. Therefore, Gd-containing nanoparticles can be used as a theragnostic agent for cancers.

Gd, Dy, Ho, Er, and Tb have large magnetic moments suitable for MRI contrast agents. Gd has a pure electron spin magnetic moment and thus ultrasmall gadolinium oxide nanoparticles can be used as a T_1 MRI contrast agent, whereas other ultrasmall lanthanide oxide nanoparticles can be used as a T_2 MRI contrast agent. Since lanthanide elements have large X-ray attenuation powers, their oxide nanoparticles can be used as a CT contrast agent. Eu and Tb strongly fluoresce in red and green regions, respectively,

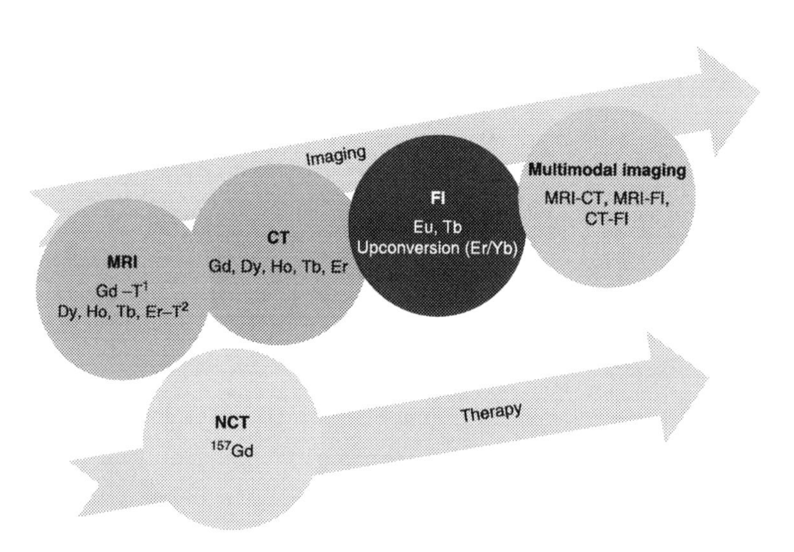

Figure 8.1 Possible application areas of ultrasmall lanthanide oxide and mixed lanthanide oxide nanoparticles to nanomedicine

and thus their oxide nanoparticles can be used as a FI agent. By combining these elements, ultrasmall mixed lanthanide oxide nanoparticles can be used as various multimodal imaging agents. These include MRI-CT, MRI-FI, CT-FI, and MRI-CT-FI, etc. Ultrasmall gadolinium oxide nanoparticles can be used as a NCT agent. Therefore, Gd-containing lanthanide oxide nanoparticles can be used for both imaging and GdNCT. Therefore, ultrasmall lanthanide oxide and mixed lanthanide oxide nanoparticles are promising materials in diagnosis and treatment in nanomedicine. Their possible application areas are schematically drawn in Figure 8.1.

8.2 What needs to be done for clinical applications

The state-of-the-art in science and technology of nanoparticles would be the clinical application of them to humans. We call this 'nanomedicine'. As already discussed, ultrasmall lanthanide oxide nanoparticles can be applied to a variety of single and multimodal imagings such as MRI, CT, FI, MRI-CT, and MRI-FI, CT-FI. In addition, ultrasmall gadolinium oxide nanoparticles can be applied to NCT.

For clinical applications, ultrasmall lanthanide oxide nanoparticles should be non-toxic (or biocompatible) and completely excreted from the body through renal system as urine. This is because ultrasmall lanthanide oxide nanoparticles are toxic and cannot be digested in the body, because there is no metabolic process to consume them. For non-toxicity, ultrasmall lanthanide oxide nanoparticles should be well-coated with a hydrophilic and biocompatible ligand. This will make them water-soluble and biocompatible while circulating in the body after intravenous injection. For renal excretion as urine, hydrodynamic diameter of ligand coated ultrasmall lanthanide oxide nanoparticles should be less than 3 nm. Otherwise, they will accumulate in the body, which would be harmful.

Index